NO-NONSENSE GUIDE TO

ANTIBIOTICS

DANGERS, BENEFITS & PROPER USE

A SmartMEDinfo Book by

Moira Dolan, M.D.

No-Nonsense Guide to Antibiotics:
Dangers, Benefits & Proper Use
A SmartMEDinfo Book
By Moira Dolan, M.D.
Copyright © 2015 by Moira Dolan, M.D., SmartMEDinfo

For permission requests, contact publisher through http://www.smartmedinfo.com.
Ordering Information:

Quantity sales. Special discounts are available on quantity purchases by corporations, associations, and others. Orders by U.S. trade bookstores and wholesalers. For details, contact the publisher through http://www.smartmedinfo.com.

Disclaimer:

The information provided here is an interpretation of information that is made generally available to the physician. This is not intended to be a comprehensive nor exhaustive review of everything known in any quarter about the topics and it is not medical advice. It is provided as a supplement to patient/doctor discussions in order to facilitate informed consent. Patients are advised to consult with their trusted health care practitioner if they are considering changes in their medication regimen.

Editing by The Pro Book Editor
Interior design services provided by Indie Author Publishing Services
Cover design by Alex Croft

ISBN: 978-0-9968860-2-4
Main category—Reference>Consumer Guides
Other category—Health & Fitness>Health Care Issues
Printed in the United States of America
First Edition

OTHER BOOKS

Dedicated to the memory of Dr. Albert Schweitzer. Many are glad he lived. He once said, "Man can hardly even recognize the devils of his own creation."

TABLE OF CONTENTS

CHAPTER 1

Who Needs This Book

Antibiotics are medications prescribed to treat infections caused by bacteria while other classes of drugs treat infections caused by viruses, fungus, or parasites. Antibiotics can be miraculously effective when used to combat life-threatening bacterial infections, but like all drugs, the smart health care consumer should know about their darker side.

- The Centers for Disease Control (CDC) estimates over half the antibiotics prescribed for patients who visit a clinic in the United States are inappropriate.

- Most of these patients are seeing the doctor for sore throats or colds that are in fact caused by viruses, not bacteria. [1]

- 7 of the top 15 medications involved in drug injuries are antibiotics. [2]

- Antibiotics cause 1 out of 5 emergency department visits for drug side effects, more officially termed "adverse drug events." [3]

- Antibiotics are the most frequent cause of drug reactions in children. [4]

In the US, $11,000,000,000 are spent every year on antibiotics. Antibiotic overuse is so common that the bugs are getting smarter—a critical number of bacteria have already reprogrammed their genes to become resistant to drugs. Antibiotic resistance is now officially a "global public health threat" according to the World Health Organization (WHO). [5] As reported on BBC online, the WHO report described the so-called post-antibiotic era we are entering as a time "where people die from simple infections that have been treatable for decades." [6]

A Bloomberg editorial from 2016 states, "The end of the Antibiotics Era may be nigh." [7] A Forbes writer describes "Antibiotic Apocalypse" in which two-thirds of deaths from infection could be due to antibiotic resistance. [8]

What happens if there is a terrorist attack with anthrax, but because tetracycline and Cipro have been so overused in the past they don't touch anthrax? Or, what about the more likely scenario, when common ear infections, pneumonia, or Strep throat are completely untreatable by even our big gun antibiotics?

This book outlines what you need to consider when offered a prescription for antibiotics. Smart health care consumers know it is necessary to be fully informed before ingesting medications, especially in light of how many unnecessary prescriptions are being written. At the least you should find out:

- Do you even have a bacterial infection?

- How well does the drug work for your specific condition?

- What is known about the antibiotic's side effects?

- What are the alternatives to taking an antibiotic, including the expected result if you take no medicine at all? (Even when the infection is bacterial, most people with healthy immune systems fight off an infection on their own.)

In fact, your prescribing doctor is ethically and legally obligated to inform you of all of these points, but this is almost never done. You have a right to full Informed Consent, meaning the right to be told all the facts so that you can logically decide whether or not to accept the risks that come with taking medication. If this is not done, you could really be in for some serious yet preventable, even unnecessary, drug side effects.

Per the official legal definition, Informed Consent requires the patient be in possession of their faculties, meaning not mentally incompetent. In today's health care system, it is almost never mental incompetence inhibiting rational medical decision-making. [9] Some patients may feel social pressures, ridicule, or financial pressures; or fear being labelled "non-compliant" for not following doctor's orders or questioning popular medical trends. The usual seven-minute patient-doctor face-to-face visit can also prevent the opportunity for real informed consent.

But most of the time, lack of informed consent is because of a combination of ignorance and low ethics. Sadly, most patients do not know about their legal right to informed consent and most physicians feel no ethical responsibility to provide it. Doctors in a busy practice don't go home and read medical journals about the actual facts, figures, and side effects of drugs, and rarely ever with a critical eye if they do. Most do not challenge the latest drug news supplied by pharmaceutical marketing divisions, but rather depend on the steady stream of drug company promotional material to tell them what treatments they should offer.

The Western tradition of medical ethics dates back to Hippocrates, a Greek physician from about 500 BC. His writings are the earliest Greek medical documents known and include the famous Hippocratic Oath. There are many translations of what is believed to be the original oath scribed by Hippocrates. Classical versions are an oath to the gods and include promises to honor one's teacher, pass on one's medical knowledge, apply nutritional remedies, refrain from using or suggesting deadly drugs, refuse to participate in abortion, leave surgery to the surgeons, maintain patient confidentiality, and never engage in sexual relations with a patient. It is generally interpreted as simply keeping the patient's best interests at heart. [10]

It may come as a shock that medical schools do not have any requirement for graduating doctors to take any oath. When the Oath is read at an optional convocation ceremony, most have taken the liberty of modifying the original. Popular revisions include dropping the opening vow to the gods, omitting any reference to prohibition against abortion, and qualifying the ban on sexual activity with patients. In short, this ethical guide has been dropped or watered down to fit modern morals, or amorality, as the case may be.

The Oath has been popularly summarized as meaning "first do no harm," which is a phrase that does not actually appear in the classical version. The promise to refrain from using deadly drugs is the true predecessor to informed consent.

Knowing all drugs have some potential for adverse effects, how does the modern day physician adhere to an oath to refrain from giving or suggesting deadly drugs? The practice of providing informed consent is the closest medical practitioners come to really applying the ethical code the oath is meant to represent. Unfortunately, most physicians don't genuinely give the opportunity for informed consent despite national guidelines, state level legislation, and medical board policies that require informed consent to varying degrees.

This book is for parents who want to do the right thing for their children, adults caring for physically vulnerable elderly family members, spouses who are looking after the best interest of their loved ones, and smart health care consumers who suspect they are not getting enough information from their doctor. And it would do some good for nurse practitioners, physician assistants, and doctors to read it, too!

The *No-Nonsense* series gives information on drugs often not shared by your doctor and not easy to extract from Internet sources. This material is an interpretation of information on the more common antibiotics prescribed in an out-patient setting. Although the data in this book is readily available to physicians, they often fail to stay informed and almost never help their patients weigh risks versus benefits when issuing antibiotic prescriptions. Use this book as a supplement to patient/doctor discussions in order to facilitate informed consent.

This is not intended to be a comprehensive nor exhaustive review of everything known in any quarter about all antibiotics. For example, it does not address most of the intravenous antibiotics given to severely ill patients in the intensive care unit. In that setting, the immediately life-threatening nature of the infection obviously outweighs concern about potential drug side effects.

On the other end of the risk/benefit spectrum, humans shouldn't expect perfect health or a wonder drug to instantly restore it. In between, you will find situations that call for a careful consideration of the need for and choice of antibiotics. You are now on your way to being a smart health care consumer.

CHAPTER 2

ANTIBIOTIC RESISTANCE

A strain of bacteria is "resistant" when it can live in high concentrations of an antibiotic. Survival of the fittest: bacteria are forced to develop resistance after being repeatedly exposed to an antibiotic. Only the bacteria that have some biochemical quirk or mutant genetic makeup can survive, and then the new, resistant bacteria make more generations like themselves. These survivor strains can function and persist when other strains are dying off from antibiotic treatment. The more widespread the use of antibiotics, the greater the numbers of individual bacteria that are exposed to threats and compelled to develop survival tactics.

Bacteria have several avenues of developing resistance. They can change their DNA to modify the shape of the receptors on their surfaces, sort of like changing out the lock so the key (the drug) no longer fits and cannot gain access. Bacteria can modify their internal metabolism so that they skirt around the points disrupted by antibiotics. They can develop more effective mechanisms for pumping antibiotics out of themselves, reducing the concentration of poison inside. They can also modify the drug molecule to make it inactive.

Bacterial DNA is changed by mutation of existing genes, or by snagging new genes from the environment. New genes can come from the act of "conjugation"—a sort of bacterial sex that allows swapping of gene particles. Viruses that infect the bacteria can carry new genes in. Some genetic elements that code for antibiotic resistance are free-floating in the environment. At least one study has shown the presence of antibiotic drugs alone is enough to trigger bacteria to ingest these submicroscopic pieces of genes and incorporate them permanently into their own DNA. [1]

These numbers show just how bacteria are able to stay ahead of new antibiotic drug development:

- Bacteria have been evolving on Earth one thousand times longer than man.

- Bacteria are about 10 sextillion times more numerous than humans (that's 10 to the 22nd power; 10,000,000,000,000,000,000,000 times more).

- Bacteria produce new generations every 30 minutes on average, while we make a new generation roughly every 30 years.

This shows that bacteria have the ability to adapt much faster and with more flexibility than the relatively slow and complex human body. [2]

The modern era of antibiotic use started in the 1930s with sulfa drugs. By 1940, antibiotic resistance to sulfa was detected. Next came penicillin, which provoked the development of resistant bacteria in just a few years. Streptomycin was used for about 15 years before resistance was detected. Tetracycline resistance emerged just a few years after its introduction. The two most recently developed antibiotics, Linezolid and Daptomycin, were associated with bacterial resistance in 4 years and 1 year, respectively. In fact, if you have taken an antibiotic recently, there is a measurable amount of antibiotic-resistant bacteria on and inside you, according to Dr. Jeffry Linder of Harvard Medical School. [3]

Increasingly, antibiotic "cures" promote the development of worse, incurable infections. The World Health Organization (WHO) regards antibiotic resistance as a "global emergency." Infection with antibiotic resistant bacteria can result in more than twice the death rate of people infected with susceptible bacteria. In its 2013 report, "Antibiotic Resistance Threats in the United States," the Centers for Disease Control (CDC) stated, "Up to half of antibiotic use in humans and much of antibiotic use in animals is unnecessary and inappropriate and makes everyone less safe." [4]

The existence of so-called superbugs was predicted, but we are only recently seeing it in horrifying real life. The first case of an E coli infection resistant to the super-drug colistin was reported in China in 2015, and by 2016, there was a case in the US. [5]

In late 2016, a Nevada woman died from an overwhelming infection caused by bacteria that were resistant to all antibiotics the hospital had, and to all known antibiotics available in the US. [6] When the bacteria circulating in her blood was grown in the lab and subjected to a series of powerful antibiotics, including colistin, it didn't even make a dent in its growth.

A gene mutation called mcr1 in the bacterium Klebsiella pneumonia was responsible for two earlier cases of death from superbugs. The mcr1 gene is getting a lot of attention because it is found in a snippet of free DNA on what is called a plasmid. The plasmid can be freely passed to other Klebsiella bacteria, but also to bacteria of other (unrelated) species.

But in the Nevada case, the bacteria did not have the mcr1 gene; some other unknown mechanism was making the bacteria untouchable by antibiotics. Survivor strains can function and persist when other strains are dying off from antibiotic treatment. The more widespread the use of antibiotics, the greater the numbers of individual bacteria that are exposed to threats and compelled to develop survival tactics.

Some genetic elements that code for antibiotic resistance are free-floating in the environment. At least one study has shown the presence of antibiotic drugs alone is enough to trigger bacteria to ingest these submicroscopic pieces of genes and incorporate them permanently into their own DNA.

Are you at risk of death from superbugs?

It is highly unlikely because your own baseline health and vitality are much more important than the kinds of bugs you meet. These are called "host factors," as if your body is the host to the guest bacteria. The main predictors of susceptibility to infection have to do with the host factors of proper nutrition, and freedom from underlying severe disease, as well as freedom from toxic substances that impair nutrition and the immune system. Topping the list of offending drugs are steroids, medications that inhibit stomach acid, and excessive use of antibiotics.

Let's look at some of the ways antibiotic resistance is encouraged in our society.

Unnecessary Use of Antibiotics in Humans

Four out of five Americans were prescribed an antibiotic in 2010 when there were about 309 million Americans total. That amounted to 258 million courses of drugs. More than 104 million of those were for azithromycin and amoxicillin—the most commonly prescribed. At least half of all antibiotic prescriptions were not necessary, according to the CDC, so about 130 million prescriptions should not have been written. [7]

In fact, all antibiotic package inserts plainly warn they should only be used in cases of proven or strongly suspected bacterial infection, and that giving antibiotics only for prevention is unlikely to provide benefit to the patient while increasing the risk of drug resistance.

It is extremely common practice to take antibiotics for the common cold, but that is a viral infection and therefore not affected by antibiotics at all. There are always bacterial bystanders—bacteria that are present but not causing infection or disease in any way. The susceptible bystander bacteria are killed off, leaving only the few resistant survivors that will propagate new generations, all inheriting the resistance genes. When those bacteria cause an infection, the usual antibiotics won't be effective.

Along with colds, ear infections in children are a major application of unneeded antibiotics. It is estimated that kids are prescribed antibiotics at least twice as often as they need them. Bronchitis in adults is almost always viral, and is never supposed to be treated by antibiotics unless it is a rare case of whooping cough. Non-specific fever and runny nose—called "influenza like illness" but not actually caused by influenza—is another area of profound antibiotic overuse. Of course, the true flu is a viral infection and there is likewise no role for antibiotics in most cases there, either.

Unnecessary Use of Antibacterial Chemicals

These days, public places are probably the most abundant sources of excessive antibacterial chemicals. Antibacterial hand sanitizer stations are in the mall, bank lobbies, grocery stores, schools, and airports. Here are just a few things that are treated with or contain antibacterial chemicals in your everyday environment:

semi-synthetic countertops	hairbrushes
food slicers	deodorant
kitchen towels	socks
cutting board and implements	underwear
notebooks	clothes
scissors	baby seats
plastic storage boxes	vacuum cleaners
soaps	yoga mats
toothpaste	football helmets
foundation	water coolers
lip gloss	paint
mascara	wall coverings
lotions	tile grout

The two most common antibacterial chemicals in consumer objects are triclosan and a related compound called triclocarban. Way back in 2000, the American Medical Association (AMA) stated, "Despite their recent proliferation in consumer products, the use of antimicrobial agents such as Triclosan in consumer products has not been studied extensively. No data exists to support their efficacy when used in such products or any need for them...." Indeed, these chemicals have never been proven to be more effective than good old-fashioned soap and water. The Food and Drug Administration (FDA) has concerns about hormonal effects of triclosan. In a 2013 statement, the FDA stated these antimicrobials "could pose health risks, such as bacterial resistance or hormonal effects." The FDA has cited studies showing that after a single treatment with triclosan, animals have poor function of heart and skeletal muscles. Other animal studies have found triclosan causes reduced or absent sperm and abnormalities in the cells that make sperm. [8]

In a 2010 press release, Natural Resources Defense Council (NRDC) Senior Scientist Dr. Sarah Janssen said, "With no proven benefit and many red flags raised for harmful health impacts, the use of these so-called anti-microbials is an unnecessary and stupid use of toxic chemicals." The NRDC has called on the US FDA to ban the chemical. [9]

Triclosan is intended to persist, and it does. When antibacterial wipes are used, triclosan leaves residues behind. Bacteria that change their protein structure slightly are unaffected by the drug, and emerge even stronger to multiply by the billions. Then they are washed down the drain to be widely distributed into the environment. [10] A more insidious danger of triclosan is that keeping indoor environments excessively clean gives children less to be exposed to, and fewer microorganisms for his or her young body to develop strong defenses against. Too sterile an environment could be a cause of childhood allergies and weakened immune systems.

Excessive Use of Antibiotics in Feed Animals

Human overuse of antibiotics and antibacterial agents is not the only problem. The overuse in food animals has been a cause of concern for decades longer. More than 29 million pounds of antibiotics are used in factory farms, which amounts to more than 70% by weight of antibiotics sold in the US—this is far more antibiotics than used by other nations. American food animals are given about six times as much antibiotics as are food animals in Norway and Denmark, for example. [11]

Today's animal production methods center on Confined Animal Feeding Operations (CAFOs), or factory farms, where hogs, cattle, and poultry are kept and raised in confined situations. Such close quarters are unsanitary and lead to easy spread of infection. The alternate solution pharma business recommends is to increase the use of preventative vaccines in feed animals by lacing the livestock's food and sometimes even spraying the animals with vaccines. In egg factories, for instance, eggs are sprayed with vaccines. The US Department of Agriculture licenses more than 2,000 vaccines for use in animals. Most of these vaccines are inactivated formulations, but more than a quarter of them (over 500) are live formulations—meaning live bacteria or viruses are present in the vaccine. These live vaccines could potentially transmit disease to humans. Veterinary vaccines are intended only for use in animals, therefore are not tested for safety in humans. [12]

Vaccines can be liberally used while still calling the product "organic" and "antibiotic free," so consumers may have no idea of their exposure. A report from Australia in 2012 described the use of 2 live-virus vaccines against different viruses in a chicken factory. They combined to form a new super-virus that spread like wildfire and sickened the animals. [13]

The swine flu virus is an example of how factory animal facilities can force the development of aggressive viral strains in humans. The virus has been around since the 1930s, and did not mutate much at all until 1998 when there was an outbreak of flu caused by a new strain at a pig factory in North Carolina. After that, swine flu virus became unstable and spread more easily to humans. The reason to suspect swine flu vaccine is that when all pigs are vaccinated, only the mutant resistant strains will survive. This phenomenon is called "genetic drift" and it is pressured to occur when there is heavy use of vaccinations. Of course, this is convenient for the vaccine manufacturers, because it constantly calls for new vaccines to be developed.

To make matters worse, the guts of farm animals do not break down antibiotics, so these drugs pass into their urine and feces virtually unchanged. [14] Manure is often used as fertilizer to enrich the soil of food crops. Humans eat from food crops containing resistant bacteria. In this way, antibiotic resistance grows by leaps and bounds. A more disturbing way of getting rid of factory farm waste is to drain the cesspools of animal feces and urine by pumping out the toxic liquid and spraying it into the environment. You can see a video of that process captured by a drone over a pig factory on the "factoryfarmdrones" website. [15]

Resistant bacteria can be spread in both directions, with animals getting resistant bugs passed to them through their human animal handlers and people working with livestock getting resistant bacteria from animals and dead meat they work with or eat. Aquaculture facilities (fish farms) are also heavy users of antibiotics, and the bacteria in fish use the same mechanisms to develop resistance as do bacteria in land animals. Significant concentrations of over 47 different antibiotics have been found in packaged fish from the grocery store, including in some fish labeled "antibiotic-free." [16]

If a person gets ill with one of these resistant bugs, the usual antibiotics will not work. The result could be an increased length of illness, extended hospital stay, or death. More than 75% of drugs used in feed animals are also used to treat human diseases, with six of these among the critically most important drugs in the world, and these critical drugs are fast losing their potency. [17]

Drug makers want taxpayers to fund more research and development (R&D) into new antibiotics. But a dirty, not-so-secret accounting deception by pharma is that what is counted in their R&D budget is off by some 90%. It turns out that small companies and the government (taxpayers) pay for the majority of basic science development, their figures do not deduct savings from huge tax breaks for nearly 40% of their reported R&D costs, and their cost per year for development of each drug is falsely reported over 7.5 years versus the 4-year average time it actually takes to get a drug through the FDA. [18]

If pharma wants more R&D money, they should take it from their rich marketing budgets: 9 out of the world's top 10 pharmaceutical companies far outspend on marketing drugs compared to what they spend on developing new drugs. For example, Johnson & Johnson spent $17.5 billion on marketing—more than double its $8.2 billion in R&D costs. [19]

Pharmaceutical Drug Waste

Treated water coming from any pharmaceutical company's antibiotic manufacturing plant is a source of genetic material, in that it includes organisms with genes coding for drug resistance. An analysis of the wastewater from one such facility showed that their clean-up process removed at least 80% of the drug resistant genes, leaving up to 20% potentially discharged into the environment. [20]

Another category is general pharmaceutical waste, which includes expired, unused, spilt, and contaminated pharmaceutical products, drugs, vaccines, and sera that need to be disposed of appropriately. This is all in addition to general healthcare waste that includes discarded items used in the handling of pharmaceuticals, such as bottles or boxes with residues, gloves, masks, connecting tubing, and drug vials, as well as flushed drugs and the undigested drugs in the toilets of human antibiotic users. Antibiotic resistant bacteria have been found in all tap water tested in Michigan and Ohio, and this finding has been reported in populated areas from India to Germany. Only very high temperature incineration can be relied upon to neutralize pharmaceutical drugs, but guidelines for such waste disposal are largely voluntary and irregularly applied. [21, 22]

Water Purification

It may not seem obvious to look for antibiotic resistance in water purification plants. Increasingly, large public water systems are relying on a process that uses bacteria in conjunction with activated carbon, ozone, and chlorine to prepare public drinking water. Biologically Activated Carbon (BAC) consists of carbon processed to greatly increase its surface area with man-made tiny holes and irregular surfaces. These surfaces are seeded with bacteria in a concentration of about one billion organisms per gram of carbon. The carbon is treated with ozone, which significantly enhances the biological activity of the resident bacteria. When water is passed through the carbon, some polluting chemicals get stuck onto the carbon and the bacteria go to work neutralizing the toxic chemicals. Then the water is typically treated with chlorination. A major concern with these systems is how it specifically uses chemical resistant bacteria, which causes the growth of more numerous resistant bacteria. A study of purified water from a large city purification system showed that while many genes coding for resistance were effectively filtered out, one very dangerous gene remained untouched. [23]

Studies done on city tap water have shown the growth of antibiotic resistant bacteria, with most resistant to not just one but several different kinds of antibiotics. BAC filtration, ozonation, and the byproducts of chlorination can greatly enhance the abundance of antibiotic resistance in community water.

Biofilm

Bacteria that are normally free-floating can be pressured by threats to their survival into making biofilm. The sticky substance helps bacteria latch on to host tissues and shields bacteria within a gel-like matrix where they are effectively hidden from antibiotics. It also acts as a cell-to-cell communication medium through which vital information—such as how to build resistance to the latest antibiotic—is rapidly spread. Biofilm is also known as slime, like that found in restaurant ice machines, on water pipes, and in aquariums, and may contain more than one strain of bacteria, parasites, and fungus.

Not all biofilms are bad. Some are used to clean up environmental disasters like oil spills and in water processing plants to convert waste water to safe water. Human large intestine is lined with a biofilm that keeps beneficial bacteria in place. [24]

Dental plaque is another human version of biofilm, and biofilm is always a factor in severe gum disease. It contributes to antibiotic-resistant infections such as bacterial sinus infection, chronic bacterial bronchitis, non-healing open wounds, and persistent bladder infections.

Nutritional deficiencies in the human host can drive bacteria into making biofilm. This has been studied most in mouth biofilm that accompanies chronic gum disease, which has been associated with deficiencies in antioxidants, vitamin C, vitamin D, calcium, and dietary fat (omega 3s). [25]

Treatment for the biofilm aspect of resistant infections can include digestive enzymes. Trypsin, chymotrypsin, and pancrease are the same enzymes that the pancreas uses to digest food and they can help break down tough slime associated with chronic infections. [26] Plant enzymes also work, such as bromelain from pineapples and papain from papaya. [27]

What Can Be Done About It?

Demanding informed consent from your would-be antibiotic prescriber is a way to minimize impacts from antibiotic resistance. This entails being told:

- the drug mechanism of action,

- what is known about its effectiveness (how well it works), and

- what is known and unknown about its safety.

Challenge blanket statements.

- If you are told you need an antibiotic, ask if and when the illness will resolve on its own.

- Be suspicious of providers who don't discuss the details of medication side effects or refuse to have a conversation about viable options other than antibiotic prescriptions.

- When you look up something on the Internet, click around to see if you can tell who is sponsoring the information and take into account any signs of conflict of interest when reading compelling marketing material.

- At the very least, do not take any medical advice from commercials, talk shows, TV news doctors, or NPR!

Physician education is only partially effective. There has been a plateau in the inappropriate prescribing of antibiotics to children in response to pressure from the American Academy of Pediatrics (AAP) recommended guidelines, but other national practice guidelines have not been heeded. Part of the problem is fear of lawsuits from failing to give an antibiotic when it was really needed. Malpractice concern seems greater among non-physician practitioners, who are generally more liberal with antibiotic prescriptions than are doctors. In fact, there is a strong correlation of overprescribing with the density of lawyers in the neighborhoods around doctor's offices. [28]

Decentralization of food production is a logical solution to the filthy, overcrowded conditions promoting infectious diseases among feed animals: dismantle the gigantic operations where overcrowded animals do not have room to turn around and return to smaller, dispersed animal-raising arrangements. Short of that, facilities could be kept cleaner and provided with better ventilation at the very least.

Be aware of antibiotic-laden consumer products in the environment, and avoid them whenever you have a choice.

Probably the single most effective thing people can do is adjust expectations about health and illness. A body is going to get infections, and a body with an intact immune system is going to undergo the natural process of warding off infection in the course of a short illness. We are conditioned to consider just about any illness to be unacceptable and signaling a need for drugs. In fact, signs like fever, inflammation, and even pus formation are indicators that a normal immune system is kicking in and effectively meeting the challenge of the infecting bug. Such everyday illnesses do not need medical attention, much less antibiotics.

Antibiotics can be lifesaving in certain conditions. However, for mild to moderate infections in the usually well population, patients and doctors should heed warnings against taking these drugs unless infection with bacteria is proven or strongly suspected. Obtaining sputum samples, nasal swabs, or urine samples to send for culture is worth it to avoid the human cost if we don't prevent drug side effects and antibiotic resistance.

CHAPTER 3

ANTIBIOTICS AND HUMAN ECOLOGY

"Man will ultimately destroy himself if he thoughtlessly eliminates the organisms that constitute essential links in the complex and delicate web of life of which he is a part." [1]

Renowned microbiologist René Dubos wrote these words in 1969, barely 40 years into the antibiotic era. Now, more than 40 years later, the accuracy of his prediction is plainly evident.

The human digestive tract is not only a passageway for food. The gut lining is a complex, highly regulated membrane essential for proper absorption of nutrients. The large bowel (the colon) contains trillions of bacteria—ten times more than there are cells in the body—consisting of some 40 different species. Fungi and single cell organisms called Archaea also live in the gut, but their roles are unknown. This bacterial mix is called the gut microbiome. A normal mix of gut organisms is necessary for the bowels to move food and waste. An altered microbiome can lessen the amount of energy the body extracts from food.

The gut bacteria digest carbohydrates to help produce energy for the body. The byproducts of bacterial carbohydrate metabolism are various acids that help the muscles and liver. These acids help force the elimination of cancer-causing substances through the stool. Bacteria help make the body's K and B vitamins; facilitate absorption of iron, calcium, and magnesium; metabolize fat; and neutralize foreign substances.

Normal gut bacteria stick to the lining, forming a sort of barrier that makes it harder for other bacteria or fungus to attach, overgrow, and invade to cause disease. This is an example of a beneficial biofilm. Some normal human gut bacteria secrete substances that are harmless to humans but act as poison to invading bacteria. Microbes maintain normal permeability of the gut lining so nutrients can enter the bloodstream but toxins, infectious bacteria, and viruses cannot.

There are nests of immune cells throughout the small bowel and large bowel. Normal gut bacteria stimulate the immune cells to make antibodies against germs and toxins. They 'train' the body to recognize helpful bacteria and attack bad bacteria. The normal complement of colon bacteria provides anti-inflammatory protection to the gut. The full scope of the interaction between healthy gut bacteria and the immune system is not known, but an altered bacterial composition contributes to allergies, asthma, and diseases where the immune system is attacking one's own body (autoimmune diseases). The optimal bacterial population modulates the local immunity reactions in the gut, but when there is a deficit of the correct bacteria, the bowel walls get inflamed and leaky. This lets substances seep into the bloodstream that would not normally be permitted. For example, when the leaky gut permits large protein molecules in, the body reacts by making antibodies to counter the foreign substance. In the joints, for instance, antibodies can cross-react with normal tissues, causing arthritis; or in the brain, causing fogginess.

There are more nerve cells (neurons) in the gut than in the spinal cord. There are cell surface receptors for numerous nerve-signaling biochemicals (neurotransmitters) such as dopamine, serotonin, glutamate, norepinephrine, and nitric oxide. In fact, the majority of the body's serotonin is made in the gut by use of a chemical generated by bacteria. [2]

Disruption of normal bacterial mix in the gut might well contribute to mood changes. This nervous system in the gut is now being called "the enteric nervous system" or the "gut brain." It is highly dependent on the right bacterial mix for normal functioning. [3] The gut interacts with the brain in both directions. The brain fires the vagus nerve, which in turn sends branches into the intestines. In the other direction, the gut releases chemicals that cause nerves to relay messages, called neurotransmitters, that influence the brain. The bacterial population in the gut influences the neurotransmitter release, thus affecting what messages go to the brain. Animal studies have shown that placing certain bacteria in the gut will eliminate anxiety behavior in mice. An abnormal bacteria mix can alter an animal's perception of pain, and probably has the same effect in humans. The opposite effect also occurs: psychological stressors early in animal life influence the composition of the gut microbiome, influencing susceptibility to disease as an adult. [4]

Antibiotic-associated colitis is a raging colon infection brought on by overgrowth of certain aggressive bacteria called Clostridium difficile. C difficile overgrows unchecked when the normal gut bacteria have been wiped out by antibiotic treatment. It is estimated that 1 in 5 hospitalized patients have C difficile in their stool, but many have no symptoms. In severe cases it can cause bloody diarrhea, nausea, and vomiting. When it becomes symptomatic, the usual treatment is to stop the antibiotics causing it. If that does not alleviate the symptoms, then the patient is put on specific antibiotics directed at killing C difficile, usually metronidazole or vancomycin. Up to 20% of patients have a relapse weeks or months after what was thought to be successful treatment.

Non-antibiotic treatments for antibiotic-associated colitis seems to make more sense. For instance, fecal transplant is being investigated and shows some promise. Stool from someone else is delivered to the patient by enema, bringing with it a normal bacterial load where C difficile does not predominate. Another non-drug treatment is heavy doses of beneficial bacteria in the form of probiotics. These non-drug options may be appropriate for mild cases of colitis or in severely ill people who have failed to respond to antibiotic treatment. [5]

The gut microbiome is always going to be affected to some degree when you take a course of antibiotics. To minimize the adverse effects during and after the antibiotic treatment you can take these measures:

- Maintain an acidic stomach environment by taking apple cider vinegar or Zypan (Standard Process-R).

- Take probiotics containing at least *Lactobacillus* and *Bifidobacterium.*

- Feed good bacteria with fruits and vegetables, especially pears, root vegetables, beans, jicama, asparagus, onions, garlic, and artichokes.

- Starve bad bacteria by avoiding sugar and refined grains since these specifically feed unwanted bacteria.

- Help digestion of fat with betaine, which comes from beetroot, quinoa, spinach, and wheat bran.

- Break up gut biofilm that contains damaging bacteria by eating okra and taking digestive enzymes such as pepsin, bromelain, maltase, amylase, lactase, lipase, peptidase, and proteases.

- Repair the gut lining with the amino acid glutamine taken as a supplement capsule or naturally supplied by sipping bone broth.

- Restore the lost vitamins, particularly vitamins A, E, K, and B.

- Supply beneficial yeast with the capsule form of the preferred organism *Saccharomyces boulardii.* It has been shown to regulate the correct balance of organisms in the gut microbiome, interfere with the ability of bad bacteria to colonize and infect the gut lining, modulate the local and system-wide immune responses, stabilize the gastrointestinal barrier function, and help enzymes work better to absorb and supply nutrition to the body. [6]

- Additional healing herbs may be necessary, such as aloe vera, slippery elm bark, marshmallow root, chamomile, marigold, and Spanish moss.

The occasional life-saving effects of antibiotics can be amazing, but the all-important gut microbiome is severely endangered by the casual overuse of antibiotics for mild to moderate infections, to shorten an illness the person was going to recover from anyway, or to treat something just because it 'might' be bacterial. Antibiotic manufacturers dutifully include warnings on their package inserts alerting prescribing physicians and patients that the drugs should only be used in cases of proven or strongly suspected bacterial infection, and that giving antibiotics only for prevention is unlikely to provide benefit to the patient while increasing the risk of drug resistance. Antibiotics are probably the most abused drugs in the Western world. Preserving your normal ecology is the single most compelling reason to be very conservative about antibiotic use.

Interestingly, herbal remedies have been in use for thousands of years but have never been identified as being a cause of bacterial resistance, bacterial super-infections, or infectious colitis. There are extensive compilations of antibacterial herbs, and many of the plants have impressive scientific evidence of effectiveness as good as or better than antibiotic drugs. An in-depth description of herbal alternatives is beyond the scope of this book, but these are some reputable resources for further study:

Physicians' Desk Reference for Herbal Medicines, Fourth Edition. Publisher: PDR Network, 2007

American Herbal Products Association's Botanical Safety Handbook, Second Edition, by Zoë Gardner (Editor), Michael McGuffin (Editor). Publisher: CRC Press, 2013

The Complete German Commission E Monographs: Therapeutic Guide to Herbal Medicines by Siegrid Klein, Robert Rister, and Chance Riggins. Publisher: American Botanical Council, 1998

CHAPTER 4

Do You Need Antibiotics For ...?

As you learned in earlier chapters, consumers play a role in the inappropriate use of antibiotics and development of antibiotic resistance just as do the many industries they depend on. Seeking a cure for every little thing and literally buying into the sales-at-any-cost effort behind products and services without concern for long term consequences is irresponsible, and encourages the industry to grow in the opposite direction from what is best for humans long term. Consumers can choose to be responsible for *appropriate* use of antibiotics, and in doing so, influence a shift in supply and demand that could reduce negative global impacts from antibiotic resistance. Here are the national recommendations describing when antibiotics should and should not be used for typical conditions that do not need hospitalization.

Sore Throat

Sore throat is one of the most common reasons for a doctor's visit, with nearly 7 million office appointments per year. Only about 10% of sore throats are caused by Strep, formally called "Group A Streptococcal pharyngitis." Strep is the only cause of sore throat that needs a prescription for antibiotics, but 73% of people get an antibiotic prescription anyway. There is no reason for this over-prescribing because all doctor's offices have access to very inexpensive, rapid, and reliable testing for Strep that only requires a swab of the throat and gives results within 10 minutes.

The natural course of Strep throat is for the body to heal itself, with disappearance of sore throat and fever in 3 to 5 days. It is necessary to take antibiotics for a sore throat proven to be due to Strep for prevention of the rare after effects of a Strep infection, which can include heart valve infection or kidney damage. Penicillin is the drug of choice, and is generally three times cheaper than cephalosporins. [1]

The only difficulty in deciding whom to treat with antibiotics is the case of Strep carriers whose throats are colonized with Strep even when they are not sick—the Strep bacteria live in their tissues without causing illness. So when a carrier gets a sore throat, the symptoms are probably due to a non-dangerous bacteria or a virus. The only way to know for sure if they are a carrier is to do throat swabs when they are completely well. Up to 10% of kids are Strep carriers, and it causes them no harm. Antibiotics do not eradicate a carrier state. In carriers, the Strep bacteria can live harmoniously in that person's body (like thousands of other natural bacterial strains do), without causing the slightest illness. [2]

Tummy Ache

Pain in the stomach or abdomen is a symptom, not a diagnosis. Common causes of upper abdominal pain can be acid reflux, spasm of the swallowing tube, or gallstones, although there are many less common causes. Most belly aches go away on their own and do not need the attention of a doctor.

There is only one common condition that should routinely be treated with antibiotics. Ulcers of the stomach (gastric ulcer) or first part of the small bowel (duodenal ulcer) are often associated with overgrowth of an acid-resistant bacteria called Helicobacter pylori, or simply H pylori. It can be detected by a breath test, stool sample, blood sample, or sample taken by a scope placed into the stomach. Treatment to eradicate H pylori results in a reduced chance of developing an ulcer and a better chance of healing an existing ulcer. The usual regimen is 10 to 14 days of amoxicillin and clarithromycin, often given with a drug to suppress acid secretion. [3] Alternative treatments include taking probiotics containing *Lactobacillus acidophilus.* Cranberry, licorice root, goldenseal, and chamomile can all inhibit the growth of H pylori. [4]

Although H pylori is a bacterial species that can thrive in an acidic environment, it has limits. It can grow in tissues that have a pH down to 4, and only then by hiding in a protective bubble and working constantly to expel excessively acidic hydrogen ions out of its immediate space. The normal pH of the healthy person's stomach is more like 1.5 to 3.5—since the pH is measured on a logarithmic scale, that means the normal pH is 5 to 25 times more acidic than the pH in which H pylori can grow. This is why the prevention against infection with H pylori is to maintain a normal very acidic environment in the stomach (assuring a very low stomach pH). This can be accomplished by taking diluted apple cider vinegar before each meal, or more conveniently by taking acid correcting supplement tablets—these come as brand names such as HiPep or Zypan (Standard Process). H pylori growth is most aggressive when there are other free-living microbes present in the stomach. Keeping very high (normal) stomach acidity virtually sterilizes the stomach contents and gets rid of these other species too. [5]

Colds

Antibiotics do not fight infections caused by viruses. Colds, flu, most sore throats, bronchitis, and many sinus and ear infections don't require, or respond to, antibiotics because they are viral, not bacterial. One study took 1,286 nose and throat samples from people with cold symptoms. Most of the swabs showed one of three viruses. The next 13 most common causes were also viruses. Only less than one percent of cases (0.76%) were caused by bacteria. [6]

If you end up taking antibiotics for a viral infection, it will:

- not help you feel any better,

- not help you get well sooner,

- not cure the infection, and

- not protect other people around you from getting sick.

Unnecessary antibiotics for a cold will:

- promote antibiotic resistance,

- likely cause side effects, and

- disrupt the normal bacterial makeup of your digestive tract.

Flu

The flu, or influenza, is an illness caused by a virus, not bacteria. When you hear news reports about "flu season" and numbers of people ill with "the flu," you are not actually being given true influenza numbers at all. Several years ago, the government substituted the numbers of people with "influenza-like illness," or ILI, rather than reporting only actual influenza infection. ILI is simply defined as cough and/or sore throat with fever of 100°F or greater. ILI is extremely common, with some people getting these symptoms up to 6 times a year. [7] True influenza is actually responsible for only a fraction of ILI cases.

The causes of ILI include a variety of non-influenza viruses such as rhinoviruses, coronaviruses, human respiratory syncytial virus, adenoviruses, and human parainfluenza viruses. The same kind of symptoms can be caused by HIV infection, rabies, measles, herpes, hepatitis C, or leukemia. Some bacteria can cause the symptoms of "influenza-like illness," and these include Lyme disease, bacterial meningitis, Legionella, chlamydia, mycoplasma, and Strep. Drugs can cause ILI symptoms, such as interferon drugs used to treat severe arthritis or hepatitis, bone loss drugs such as bisphosphonates, anti-fungal drugs, vaccines, and especially the influenza vaccination itself. Even withdrawal from narcotics and psychiatric drugs can cause ILI. Environmental toxins can provoke an influenza-like illness, such as exposure to paint fumes or strong perfume, pesticides and herbicides, or heavy releases of pollen or mold spores.

In general, a viral cause is more likely when the fever at onset is high, there is a watery runny nose with involvement of many body systems (patient feels crummy all over), or there is a widespread rash, and other people within the home or community are likewise ill. It is typical that a person feels comfortable in between the fever episodes in a viral illness. A viral infection is also suggested by the lack of a red throat, no pus on the tonsils, and no tenderness at lymph nodes. Sometimes a health care provider might suggest that blood count is necessary to sort out the cause of an infection, but the routine blood count does not differentiate between viral and bacterial infections.

The Rapid Influenza Diagnostic Test (RIDT) involves taking a swab of nose secretions and waiting only 30 minutes for the results. Unfortunately, it is only little better than 50% accurate in adults. A positive RIDT result means the person is likely to have influenza, but a negative result does not reliably rule out actual influenza. Another test, which checks for the presence of genetic material from the influenza virus, is faster, but typically only done at a hospital laboratory and not available in a doctor's office. The most reliable test involves sending the swab to the lab to be cultured on a Petri dish and waiting 48 hours to see what grows. The purpose of testing is to prescribe anti-viral drugs if the test is positive, but the kicker is that such drugs only work if given in the first day and a half of symptoms. Who goes to the doctor after just a day or two of symptoms? Most people do not feel the need to run to the doctor so soon. This is reasonable because in the vast majority of people, the flu is a self-limited illness that needs no treatment. Sadly, inappropriate prescribing of anti-viral meds is becoming just as rampant as inappropriate antibiotic prescribing. [8]

In other words, "influenza-like illness" is not a real diagnosis, but only a description of symptoms so vague as to be meaningless. But ILI is exactly what the Centers for Disease Control (CDC) reports weekly during flu season. In fact, only a tiny percentage of people coming to the doctor for ILI ever get tested for the true flu. Usually only the very sickest get tested, and then only during winter when there is a high flu alert; of those few, the statistic ranges greatly as to how many really have the flu: from 0% to 60%, with the average being only 14%. [9]

If someone does have influenza, they can be assured that it is not a dangerous illness in most people and symptoms will resolve in a few days with no treatment. Because influenza is not a bacterial infection, taking antibiotics unnecessarily will do more harm than good.

Antiviral medications might help less than half of the people who actually have influenza, and then only shorten the illness by about 1 day if taken in the first day or two of symptoms. Common side effects of antiviral flu medications include nausea, vomiting, diarrhea, dizziness, headache, nosebleed, eye redness, insomnia, and cough or other respiratory problems. Antiviral medications carry mandatory warnings about the potential for severe psychiatric effects, like abnormal behavior, delirium, hallucinations, agitation, anxiety, altered level of consciousness, confusion, nightmares, and delusions. Suicides have been reported, especially in children. [10]

If a person is elderly, or has a disease that seriously compromises their immune system, or are on medications that are likely to hamper their ability to fight infection, then it makes sense to do specific influenza testing. If they go to the doctor after two days, then opportunity to treat with anti-viral medications may be past, but at least if it is proven to be influenza, then they will be spared unnecessary antibiotics. It must be emphasized that the vast majority of people who get infected with the actual influenza virus either have a brief, self-limited illness that resolves with no treatment whatsoever, or they remain entirely without symptoms, their immune system taking care of the infection in the background. It is only very effective drug company advertising that convinces us any and all infections need to be squelched with medication. The smart consumer should recognize that this is not only untrue, it also leads to dangerous overuse of anti-infective drugs, be they antiviral or antibiotic.

Sinus Infection

Sinusitis can happen when fluid builds up in the sinus cavities. In adults, sinus infections are caused by viruses in 9 out of 10 cases. In children, viruses are responsible in 5 to 7 out of every 10 cases. Even chronic sinusitis (with symptoms lasting longer than 8 weeks) is not usually bacterial. Other causes of fluid buildup are allergies, breathing second hand smoke or other pollutants, and nasal polyps. Children are more prone to sinus infections if they use a pacifier or drink from the bottle while lying down.

A study reported in the *Journal of the American Medical Association* reported that neither antibiotics nor nasal steroid sprays are effective for treating sinusitis. [11] Most patients who have sinus infection improve on their own within a week or two, without any antibiotics. Treating with an antibiotic only shortens the length of their discomfort by 15%, or 1-2 days.

Antibiotic guidance for sinusitis comes from the Centers for Disease Control (CDC) [12]:

- People with mild sinusitis symptoms can use over the counter remedies, but should avoid antibiotics.

- Patients with more severe or longer lasting symptoms might or might not benefit from antibiotics. Medical studies don't give strong evidence that antibiotics add much benefit.

- When antibiotics are decided upon, amoxicillin kills the two main bacteria associated with sinus infection. Broad-spectrum antibiotics are not necessary.

Over the counter or herbal decongestants or the use of a neti pot may help with symptoms. Neti is from a Sanskrit word meaning 'nasal cleansing'—this small pot has a long narrow spout that is used to pour sterile or distilled water into the nose, sometimes with salt added. Some people swear this helps, while others only experience choking and sputtering.

Ear Infection

Ear infection is almost entirely a childhood disease. Until the skull is fully formed, the tube that drains the ear into the nasal cavity (the Eustachian tube) is more horizontal than slanted downward as it is in adulthood. Thus the child's ear does not drain as well, and fluid can more easily build up. This allows germs to grow, but also promotes inflammation even when there isn't any actual bacterial or viral infection.

Middle ear infection is likely when a child has ear pain and the exam shows a bulging eardrum and fluid behind the eardrum, or there is fluid leaking out of the ear. Kids without a definite finding of fluid behind the eardrum should not be diagnosed with an ear infection.

According to the American Academy of Pediatrics (AAP) [13]:

- Antibiotic treatment is called for in infants under 6 months old when there is pain and bulging of one or both eardrums; fluid along with fever, irritability, crying and pulling on the affected ear are signs of pain in an infant.

- In children over 6 months, the AAP recommends antibiotics only if the symptoms are on both sides or if they are severe: the pain must be present for at least 48 hours, bulging must be severe, and the fever should be 102.2°F or higher.

- For children over 2 years old who have mild symptoms, parents and doctors can opt for just waiting another 2 or 3 days to see if symptoms worsen or get better on their own.

This is not to make the child suffer, but because lesser symptoms for shorter duration, especially without any fluid behind the eardrum, are not likely to be caused by bacteria. Those symptoms indicate it could be a viral infection, allergies, or just inflammation. In those instances, antibiotics are useless and can be dangerous. As described in Chapter 3, the frequent use of antibiotics in children significantly alters the natural microbes in the gut and this can have a negative impact on the immune system of those kids when they become adults.

When the decision to prescribe an antibiotic for ear infection has been made, the drug of choice is amoxicillin. The only exceptions for using a stronger drug are:

- if the child has already been on antibiotics in the preceding month, or

- if the child is allergic to amoxicillin, or

- the child also has eye infection (conjunctivitis), or

- the child has had recurrent middle ear infections that did not improve with amoxicillin.

Doctors should not prescribe antibiotics in an attempt to prevent ear infections—this only promotes the growth of antibiotic-resistant bugs and makes it that much harder to treat the next true infection.

Some kids suffer from frequent ear infections (and some adults get frequent sinus infections). A high frequency of infection calls for a closer look at diet. A major inhibitor of infection fighting capability is sugar in the diet—within half an hour of a high sugar load, the activity of infection fighting cells drops dramatically. Another dietary culprit is mucus-producing foods, which can create a more or less constant buildup of mucus in the Eustachian tube that goes from the ear to the sinuses. This creates a comfy breeding ground for bacteria, and also makes it hard for antibiotics to penetrate into the mucus matrix to get at the bacteria. Milk and related dairy products are the top offenders, but you may not suspect that wheat, potatoes, and bananas are also mucus-generators, along with processed foods, saturated fats, and some meats. In a well-intentioned effort to give their children probiotics by feeding them sweetened yogurt, parents may be making the kids more prone to infection because of the mucous-producing dairy along with the immune-suppressing sugar. A parent can limit their child's sensitivity to infection by keeping up a modest exercise program, maintaining a regular sleep schedule, and avoiding dairy and sugar.

Dental Conditions

Preventive antibiotics are recommended for people getting dental work who have a heart valve problem, mechanical valve, an artificial joint, or other implanted device. Simple cavities do not need antibiotics, but only need cleaning out of the infected material and a filling. Deep infection of the tooth pulp can sometimes require a root canal or removal of the tooth, and most dentists will also prescribe antibiotics. Similarly, short-term inflammation of the gums does not need antibiotics and can be addressed by mechanical scraping and deep cleaning. In severe cases of mouth-wide gum inflammation, oral antibiotics may be needed with several sessions of cutting away of the infected gum tissue.

Pink Eye

Irritated eyes are usually caused by a superficial viral infection or by allergies, and these conditions do not respond to antibiotics. A common diagnosis in the pediatrician's office is "pink eye," medically called conjunctivitis. The eyes may weep or ooze a sticky liquid, become itchy or burn, and get stuck shut when sleeping. When pink eye is caused by an infection, it can spread easily. Usually, people catch it from touching something that touched an infected person's eye. When it is a viral infection, pink eye is highly contagious, and family or playmates can get it from the other person's hands, pillowcases, towels, or clothes.

Morning crusting followed by watery eyes throughout the day are typical of allergies and viral infections, but can also be a sign of dry eyes. Scratchiness, grittiness, and itching of the eyes is probably caused by a virus, allergies, or dry eyes. Most cases clear on their own, without treatment. If the fluid is very thick and cloudy, the doctor may be concerned about the possibility of bacterial conjunctivitis and prescribe antibiotic drops, but the average viral eye infection cannot be helped by antibiotic eye drops.

Bronchitis

Bronchitis is inflammation of the large air passages (bronchi) due to infection. Almost all episodes of bronchitis are caused by viruses, making antibiotic prescriptions inappropriate. In fact, the American College of Physicians and the Centers for Disease Control and Prevention (CDC) both state unequivocally that whooping cough (pertussis) is the only indication for antibiotics in the treatment of acute bronchitis. It is estimated there are 8.7 million cases of bronchitis diagnosed per year in adults in the US, with less than one-half of 1% of those being pertussis. Pertussis is rare, but it can be easily diagnosed by a sputum culture and treated with appropriate antibiotics such as azithromycin, erythromycin or clarithromycin. [14]

Most cases of pertussis are very mild. It is only likely to cause a severe illness in the very young, not in adults. [15] Yet, 60% or more of people getting a bronchitis diagnosis are given an antibiotic. This distinguishes bronchitis as the most inappropriately treated of all common conditions.

What's worse is that more than half of those prescriptions are for broad spectrum antibiotics to attack a very wide variety of bacteria. The tendency of healthcare practitioners to prescribe broad spectrum antibiotics has more than doubled in the last ten years. The use of broad spectrum antibiotics instead of a drug narrowly directed at only the bacteria present strongly promotes bacterial resistance. [16,17]

What is causing inappropriate antibiotic prescribing? It could be something as simple as the time of day. A study of almost 22,000 respiratory infection visits to clinics showed that in the last hour, doctors were 26% more likely to give an antibiotic than they were in their first hour on shift. This phenomenon is called "decision fatigue"—the more tired they become, the more likely doctors just hand out prescriptions without thoughtful consideration of whether they are really needed. [18] Also, some studies show that non-physician providers like nurse practitioners and physician assistants are more likely to inappropriately prescribe antibiotics. [19] In addition, the intense use of direct to consumer advertising has had its intended effect—consumers are now asking for drugs by name for conditions they have self-diagnosed from TV or Internet ads. [20]

Pneumonia

Pneumonia is a lung infection, usually caused by bacteria. Therefore, antibiotics are almost always appropriate. There are three classifications of pneumonia depending on how the person became ill.

In community-acquired pneumonia, the person caught a bug at work or home. Most cases of community-acquired pneumonia can be outpatient treated with a shot in the doctor's office or antibiotics by mouth. If the patient is elderly or has other serious illnesses, then they should be treated in the hospital.

Hospital-acquired and healthcare associated pneumonias are more serious, as the infections are likely to be due to bacteria that are resistant to several drugs and will be harder to treat, almost always requiring more than one antibiotic and treatment for a longer time period. [21]

Lower Abdominal Pain

Lower abdominal pain could be due to constipation, stretching of dilated loops of bowel from excess gas, or food poisoning. Gynecologic conditions and kidney stones are other likely causes of lower belly pain. There are three common conditions that present with lower abdominal pain and might need antibiotic treatment: appendicitis, diverticulitis, and antibiotic-associated colitis.

Appendicitis is an inflammation of the pouch (the appendix) located at the end of the small bowel as it transitions into the colon. The standard of care in the US is to operate on all suspected cases of appendicitis in order to prevent the complications of a burst appendix. This aggressive approach results in 10 to 20% of all appendix operations being done on normal appendixes—in other words, 1 to 2 in 10 people didn't really need the operation. In some of those cases, the doctor should have just put the patient on antibiotics while carefully monitoring for any signs of worsening. It is estimated that up to 6% of those non-operated patients will have a recurrent attack and eventually need the appendix removed, but that means most of them will not and can avoid surgery by taking antibiotics. [22]

A diverticulum is an unnatural sac-like protrusion of the colon wall. It is not certain what causes these protrusions, but a low fiber diet and correspondingly less bulky stool may result in greater pressure on the gut lining to push the stool through the colon, eventually weakening the colon wall. Another theory is chronic gut wall inflammation develops from consuming inflammatory foods, and yet another factor might be chronic low level infection. Acute diverticulitis is inflammation of the sacs thought to be due to micro-perforations (holes) in diverticula (plural form of diverticulum). Diverticulitis can resolve on its own with no treatment, especially in patients who don't have a persistent fever. Diverticulitis can also progress to the point where it causes blockage of the bowel, abscess, burst bowel, or opening of passageways (fistula tracts) to other loops of bowel or other organs. If pain is severe or persistent, or fever persists, then antibiotic treatment is necessary. At this point, usually more than one drug is required. Typical regimens include a quinolone with metronidazole, amoxicillin-clavulanate, or trimethoprim-sulfamethoxazole with metronidazole. [23]

Genital and Urinary Infections

Bladder infection, also called urinary tract infection (UTI) is common in women. It causes painful, frequent urination; urgency; and blood in the urine, sometimes with pain in the bladder. It might resolve without specific treatment. The risk of no treatment is that the infection can climb up to the kidneys, which can be severe and result in hospitalization. Antibiotics for UTI in women could include a quinolone drug (although side effects can be severe and antibiotic resistance is a strong possibility), or nitrofurantoin, which is problematic because of the potential for severe side effects, or trimethoprim-sulfamethoxazole (TMP-SMX), or trimethoprim alone if there is a sulfa allergy.

In men, nitrofurantoin is not used, as the drug does not penetrate their bladder tissues as well. In male UTIs, it is necessary to continue the TMP-SMX or a quinolone for 7 to 10 days. Again, quinolone side effects can be quite severe. When a man has symptoms of a UTI, a urethral swab should be taken to test for STDs, especially chlamydia and gonorrhea. A rectal exam should be done to see if there is inflammation of the prostate (prostatitis).

When the elderly get UTIs, they might not experience the usual symptoms. In many cases, the bladder in an elderly person is colonized with bacteria that, while abnormal, are not causing a problem. The Infectious Diseases Society of America (IDSA) has advised that elderly only get UTIs treated if they have at least 3 of these 5 criteria:

- a fever;

- increased frequency or urgency of urination, or burning when urinating;

- pain behind or near the bladder;

- a change in the smell or appearance of urine;

- a deteriorating function or mental state. [24]

A bladder infection that has spread to the upper urinary tract results in kidney infection. Signs of kidney infection are fever, flank pain, nausea, and vomiting. It is much more serious than a bladder infection, and often calls for observation in a hospital setting for 12 to 24 hours while IV antibiotic treatment is started, and then continuation of antibiotics for 10 days to 2 weeks at home.

Unsweetened cranberry juice can be effective in preventing a full-blown UTI, especially if taken at the first symptoms of urinary frequency or urgency. The active ingredient in cranberry is a non-sweet sugar called D-mannose, which makes bacteria less able to stick to the bladder wall. [25] D-mannose can be conveniently taken in tablet form, and it is often supplied in combination with white willow bark that provides pain relief from urinary burning. A teaspoon of baking soda dissolved in a cup of water also decreases urinary acidity and can help with symptoms, providing the patient does not also have a kidney stone causing the pain. Supplements that decrease the body's production of ammonia can prevent and treat UTIs. Examples include the amino acid L-arginine or products containing the enzyme arginase. (Note that arginine should be avoided by those who suffer with recurrent genital herpes.)

It is very common for persons who get frequent UTIs to also suffer from an overgrowth of *Candida*—a type of fungus normally only present in trace amounts. *Candida* overgrows and becomes invasive into tissues when there has been a long-standing disturbance of the body's normal acid-base balance, and/or the normal mix of gut microbes has been altered due to high stomach pH or antibiotics, and/or a high sugar diet has been feeding the *Candida* organisms—this includes too many sweets, starchy foods, or alcohol. A natural anti-*Candida* regimen is beyond the scope of this book, but can be found at http://www.thecandidadiet.com/candida-diet.htm. Supplementation with vitamin D3 may also prevent UTIs. [26]

Vaginal yeast infections are common but usually asymptomatic or cause only mild discomfort. *Candida albicans* is a yeast organism that is part of the normal vaginal environment, but when it overgrows, it can cause burning, redness, swelling and intense itching, and pain on intercourse, or pain on urination. There is sometimes a thick white discharge with no odor to it. A common cause of *Candida* overgrowth is prior use of antibiotics.

A mild case of vaginal yeast infection is treated with a single dose of fluconazole (Diflucan) by mouth. In cases where the vagina is colonized with a different yeast, *Candida glabrata*, it may be effective to treat with intra-vaginal boric acid capsules for two weeks. Some doctors prescribe suppression therapy, where fluconazole is taken once weekly for six months. When vaginal yeast infections are recurrent or severe, the conventional treatment is fluconazole in two sequential doses given three days apart. Many women seek alternatives to fluconazole because of its potential to be toxic to the liver. Alternatives include radical dietary restrictions, avoiding all grains and sugars; in other words, starving the overgrown yeast organisms from what they would normally feed on.

Bacterial vaginosis is a condition causing fishy-smelling vaginal discharge that results from a bacterial imbalance. Normally, the vagina is colonized with acid-forming lactobacilli. In vaginosis, the normal lactobacilli bacteria count has decreased, so the pH changes to less acidic. The lactobacilli are replaced by a mixture of bacteria that thrive in low-oxygen environments. Bacterial vaginosis makes it easier to get HIV infection, herpes simplex virus type 2 (HSV-2), gonorrhea, chlamydia, and trichomonas. One-third of the time, vaginosis resolves on its own. When treatment is necessary, it is with metronidazole (or tinidazole) or clindamycin administered either orally or intra-vaginally. These treatments cure 70-80% of cases, but 30% relapse within three months and half relapse within the year. Adding vaginal boric acid may help the response to antibiotics. (Note that boric acid is poisonous if taken by mouth.)

Trichomonas is a vaginal infection caused by a single celled animal-like parasite. It causes a foul smelling green discharge. The treatment is a single dose of metronidazole, which cures over 90% of cases. The sex partner needs to be treated also, even if they have no symptoms.

Pelvic inflammatory disease (PID) is an infection of the uterus, tubes, and/or ovaries and causes pelvic pain and tenderness on exam. A mixture of several different bacteria causes PID, and treatment should include antibiotics that target chlamydia and gonorrhea. Most patients can be treated with a shot followed by oral antibiotics they take at home, while 10% must be hospitalized for IV antibiotic treatment. Untreated PID can result in infertility, ectopic pregnancy, and chronic pelvic pain.

Syphilis, gonorrhea, and chlamydia are bacterial sexually transmitted diseases that can have severe late effects if not treated early. Syphilis can affect heart valves and the brain and can cause dementia, gonorrhea can infect the joints, and all three can cause PID. The choice of antibiotics depends on the bacterial culture showing which drug it is sensitive to.

The diseases addressed above are the most common bacterial genital and urinary infections. There is no role for antibiotics in the treatment of viral infections, such as genital warts caused by human papilloma virus, herpes, molluscum contagiosum, or HIV infection.

Skin Infection

Cellulitis and erysipelas are skin infections that cause areas of redness, swelling, and warmth. Erysipelas involves the upper layer of skin and superficial lymph drainage, whereas cellulitis involves the deeper skin structures and fat. Mild cases can be treated with oral antibiotics that target killing *Streptococcus* and *Staphylococcus* bacteria. If the skin does not improve or worsens in 2 to 3 days, IV antibiotics must be used. If cellulitis is left untreated, it can progress to life threatening conditions such as necrotizing fasciitis—a deep infection that results in progressive destruction of the muscle connective tissue. Another type of infection that starts with cellulitis is toxic shock syndrome, which causes skin sloughing and high fever with shock and delirium or coma. Gas gangrene can occur after trauma to a limb or in diabetics. It is a foul-smelling infection that kills tissue rapidly. [27]

A common skin infection in children is impetigo. It is a superficial bacterial skin infection caused by Strep or Staph. When it is confined to a small area, it can be treated with topical antibiotics. When impetigo has widely spread or is severe with fluid filled vesicles or crusty ulcers, it needs to be treated with oral antibiotics.

Wounds from bites (human or animal) should be well cleaned to remove dead tissue and blood clots. They are not usually stitched closed unless they are on the face. The Infectious Diseases Society of America recommends antibiotics in all cases of human bites to prevent infection, even though clinical studies do not support that they are really needed when the bites only involve the top layer of skin. Bites from dogs, cats, and rodents can be mild and heal on their own. Severe, deep bites need antibiotics and sometimes surgery. The usual treatments are penicillin, or amoxicillin with clavulanate (Augmentin). Cat scratch disease is a bacterial infection from bacteria transmitted by fleas. It can cause painful enlarged lymph nodes in humans, even though the cat does not get ill from carrying the infecting bacteria. Most people clear the infection on their own, but sometimes antibiotics are required (usually with azithromycin or doxycycline).

A skin abscess is a collection of pus in deeper skin tissues. It is called a boil, or furuncle when the abscess forms from a hair follicle. Several boils lumped together into a single inflammatory mass is called a carbuncle. Most skin abscesses are from bacteria, but some can be from irritating substances such as oils injected by body builders or impurities injected by IV drug users. About 75% of skin abscesses are due to the *Staphylococcus* organism and can be treated by slitting them open to allow them to drain.

Antibiotic treatment is necessary if draining does not resolve the abscess or if the patient is at risk for the infection to spread to the heart valves (in persons with pre-existing heart valve defects) or to the bones (for instance, in children with sickle cell anemia) or to the brain or lungs in patients with poor immunity (such as in kids on chemotherapy). The usual treatment is penicillin or a penicillin derivative for one week. Abscesses around the mouth, vaginal area, and rectal area are due to a mixture of many different microorganisms and require broader antibiotic treatment. Persistent abscesses should get cultured to see if there is any *methicillin-resistant Staphylococcus aureus* (MRSA). The Infectious Diseases Society of America issues regularly updated guidance on what type of MRSA infections need antibiotics.

Hidradenitis (hidradenitis supperativa) is a special case of boils. It is also called acne inversa, meaning inverted acne. Keratin is a waxy to hard substance that helps give strength to hair and nails, but when excessively produced, it blocks hair follicles and prevents them from normally shedding. Excess keratin production blocks hair follicles in moist areas like armpits, under the breasts, groin, and rectal area. Hidradenitis is not routinely treated with antibiotics unless there is secondary infection of other structures besides hair follicles. [28]

Rosacea is redness across the cheeks and nose that can be mild, or can involve tender, fluid filled bumps (pustules), or can be the extreme type that gives a knobby, red bulbous nose. The cause is not known, but it does not appear to be due to infection. Mild rosacea can be controlled by avoiding things that cause a flare, such as extremes of temperature, direct sunlight, spicy foods, alcohol, physical stress and mental stress, menopausal hot flashes, and certain medications (especially steroids or any drugs that dilate veins). The first line of drug treatment is to try anti-inflammatory drugs on the skin (metronidazole, azelaic acid, topical ivermectin, or sulfacetamide-sulfur). More severe rosacea can be treated with tetracycline on the skin; a combination of benzoyl peroxide with clindamycin or erythromycin can be tried. If topical treatment fails, then oral antibiotics may be necessary. The usual drug is a tetracycline (doxycycline or minocycline) or clarithromycin. There does not seem to be a bacterial infection in rosacea, but these drugs are thought to work because they are anti-inflammatory. [29]

Methicillin-resistant Staphylococcus aureus (MRSA) is the main "superbug" that is resistant to antibiotics. It was rare 30 years ago, but now it is the infecting organism in some 60% of skin infections seen in a typical emergency room. The treatment of very ill hospitalized patients with MRSA is intravenous vancomycin, but antibiotics are not always necessary in people who have healthy immune systems. Cleaning and normal wound care may be all that is necessary. The best prevention against MRSA is good hand washing habits. [30]

CHAPTER 5

TRAVELER'S DIARRHEA

Diarrhea while on vacation or business travel is no fun, but for Westerners, it rarely results in hospitalization. Technically, it's an inconvenient but natural part of imperfection in our bodies and environment. Traveler's diarrhea usually begins in the first week of travel and resolves on its own within 3 to 5 days.

- Only 5 to 10% of those with traveler's diarrhea will get true dysentery with blood in the stool, fever, and chills.

- Between 8% and 15% of affected travelers are symptomatic for longer than a week.

- About 2% develop chronic diarrhea that lasts for 1 month or more.

- Traveler's diarrhea can cause a flare of irritable bowel syndrome (IBS) in people who already have it.

- It very rarely causes death in previously healthy people, and usually only if they do not have access to clean water.

Decisions about how to prepare for and react to traveler's diarrhea should be based on expected risks. Look at the country, the food and water you will be consuming, the expected sources of contamination, and the medical conditions you already have. [1]

Where Are You Going?

The Centers for Disease Control (CDC) maintains a traveler's advisory website that provides the most up-to-date information on countries of concern: http://wwwnc.cdc.gov/travel/page/travelers-diarrhea.

Here are some general guidelines:

- Low risk destinations with attack rates of under 5% are the United States, Canada, northern European countries, England, Australia, New Zealand, Japan, and most Caribbean islands.

- Intermediate risk countries with attack rates of 8% to 20% are China, Southern Europe, Israel, South Africa, Russia, and some Caribbean islands such as Haiti and Dominican Republic.

- High-risk destinations where the attack rates range from 20% up to 75% include the developing regions of Latin America, most of Africa, Asia, and parts of the Middle East.

What Are You Consuming?

High-risk foods and drinks include:

- Uncooked vegetables

- Unpeeled fresh fruit

- Salads

- Raw or undercooked meat

- Raw or undercooked seafood (especially shellfish)

- Tap water

- Re-bottled water (check the seal)

- Ice

- Unpasteurized milk

Where Are You Eating?

Meals eaten in a private home are less risky than those eaten in a restaurant. Food from street vendors is higher risk than restaurant food, but expensiveness of restaurant does not have any correlation with protection against diarrhea.

What Are Your Medical Risks?

People who take drugs to inhibit stomach acid are at much greater risk of traveler's diarrhea because stomach acid is your first, very effective means to stop common viruses and bacteria. This defense mechanism is totally disabled when acid is reduced. These include antacids (Maalox, Mylanta, Rolaids, and Tums), acid-reducing drugs known as H2 blockers (Tagamet, Pepcid, Axid, Zantac), or the proton pump inhibitors (Prilosec, Prevacid, Zegerid, Nexium, Protonix). In one study, people on omeprazole had a 10 times greater chance of getting infected by the bacteria Campylobacter. [2] If people on these drugs have to resort to antibiotics for traveler's diarrhea, they are also at much greater risk to get antibiotic-associated colitis. [3]

People who already have a condition that compromises their immune system are at greater risk for infection. This includes those receiving chemotherapy, steroids, immune-suppressant drugs after an organ transplant or for an autoimmune condition, and those with HIV infection.

Causes of Traveler's Diarrhea

Traveler's diarrhea is caused by bacteria in more than 80% of cases, the majority due to E coli, especially in Latin American countries. A common cause is a strain of E coli that produces a toxin. The toxin secreted by enterotoxic E coli (ETEC) causes the gut cells to pour out fluids, causing diarrhea, inflammation, and cell death. ETEC is the most common cause of diarrhea in travelers to Latin America, whereas Campylobacter is relatively more common in Southeast Asia, particularly Thailand.

Cholera is a common bacterial cause of diarrhea in regions with poor sanitation, crowding, war, and famine. The bacteria Vibrio cholera produces a toxin that causes huge volumes of watery diarrhea along with vomiting. It can be deadly if the patient does not have access to clean water so they can keep ahead of dehydration. In severe cases, an IV of water, salt, and potassium is needed. Replacement of lost fluids is more important than treatment with an antibiotic.

Viruses cause from 2% to 27% of traveler's diarrhea. Infection with Norovirus can happen at home, accounting for over 20 million cases a year in the US. If you hear of a viral outbreak on a cruise ship, then Norovirus is probably the culprit. A viral infection can occur in the same person who has bacterial diarrhea.

Parasites such as worms and amoeba can cause traveler's diarrhea, and parasitic infection is more likely after a prolonged out of country stay. Long lasting diarrhea (over 1 month) is particularly associated with protozoan causes of infection. Some common parasites include the tiny organisms with whip-like tails, Giardia lamblia and Dientamoeba fragilis, which can be ingested from drinking contaminated water, and also transmitted from feces that accidentally get ingested from poor hand washing. Entamoeba histolytica comes from contaminated food and water. In addition to the usual symptoms of cramping, pain, bloating, and diarrhea, it can cause infected boils on the liver. Cryptosporidium parvum can come from drinking water or going for a dip in a polluted swimming pool.

Prevention

Vaccination is only available for cholera and ETEC. The vaccine contains several strains of cholera bacteria that have been chemically treated, thus they are inactivated. The theory is that the inactivated bacteria will be recognized by the body and provoke it into making protective antibodies so that when real live Vibrio cholera shows up, the body already has an army of antibodies ready to attack it. The vaccine also contains some treated cholera toxin, which has a chemical structure similar to ETEC toxin so the vaccine gives some protection against both of these bacterial causes of diarrhea. The vaccine is taken prior to travel, as a liquid, in two doses one week apart. The main side effects are gastrointestinal, meaning nausea, vomiting, and diarrhea—exactly the things it was supposed to prevent.

To prevent drinking contaminated water, boil it for one minute, or for three minutes if you are more than 6500 feet above sea level. Always check the seals on bottled water. Alternately, you can add iodine drops or peroxide tablets to tap water, but this may not be sufficient to kill all parasites. Avoid eating salads and raw vegetables. Fruit, including tomatoes, should be peeled, unless it has been washed thoroughly in safe water. Watermelons still carry some risk since they may be injected with water to increase their weight and selling price. Meats and fish should be thoroughly cooked, and recently—avoid pre-cooked food. It is best to avoid leftovers and condiments from previously opened bottles.

The simplest and least toxic substance to prevent traveler's diarrhea is a probiotic containing the beneficial bacteria called *Lactobacillus*, with some studies reporting a protection rate of 47%.

The over-the-counter drug bismuth subsalicylate (Pepto-Bismol) can be taken as a preventative—two tablets four times a day with food. One study showed this decreased the attack rate from 40% down to 14%. Pepto-Bismol not only can kill some bacteria, it prevents the gut cells from over-secreting liquid and quiets down inflammation. It is important to know that Pepto can blacken the mouth and turn the stool black. It is not safe for young children, those with kidney disease, or anyone who is allergic to aspirin. It is for short-term use only. It interferes with the absorption of many other drugs, including tetracycline or other antibiotics that a traveler may be taking to prevent malaria, and should not be taken by people on blood thinners or shortly after the inhaled flu vaccine.

Antibiotics can do a very good job of preventing traveler's diarrhea, reducing the incidence by 80 to 90%. However, they are only recommended for people who have particular increased risks of severe illness or death if they should get an infection—like those with cancer, HIV infection, or taking immune suppressant drugs; people with inflammatory bowel disease, insulin-dependent diabetes, or those on diuretics (water pills). Unnecessary use of antibiotics forces bacteria to develop resistance and if the person should become infected, the usual antibiotics might not work. Worse, one person's resistant bugs can easily spread to others.

There is a great deal of antibiotic resistance after several decades of preventively using doxycycline or the combination drug trimethoprim-sulfamethoxazole (TMP-SMX, Septra). Fluoroquinolones are often recommended, but their mental side effects and tendon-injuring effects make these a poor choice for a preventive drug. Resistance to this class of drug is also growing, and they are practically useless in Southeast Asia. Alternate antibiotics such as azithromycin (Zithromax) and rifaximin are less well studied, and antibiotic resistance is growing to these agents, too.

Treatment of Diarrhea

Before considering antibiotics to treat diarrhea, remember that it is a self-limiting condition—you are expected to recover as long as you can keep up with your losses of fluids and electrolytes. Make your own recovery drink by adding one teaspoon of table salt and eight teaspoons of sugar to one liter of boiled or bottled water. Alternately, there are many brands of powdered re-hydration salt packets; preparations that also contain rice powder or some other form of easily absorbable sugar are more effective.

Loperimide (Imodium) can be taken to slow down or stop diarrhea. It is an opioid drug related to morphine, but available without prescription because it does not get absorbed very well, tending to stay within the bowel. It works by slowing down the internal muscular contraction of the intestines. Loperimide can be dangerous in some situations. Some diarrheal bacteria make the colon lining more permeable, in which case loperimide may enter the blood stream and cause more mental side effects. It should not be used when there is fever or blood in the stool. It should not be used by people with liver problems or while drinking heavily on vacation.

If you resort to antibiotics to treat diarrhea, follow the dosing instructions.

Antibiotics taken while traveling should be purchased at home and brought along. This will assure you do not purchase some unknown or dangerous drug in a foreign country, such as chloramphenicol or chlorhydroxyquin—both of which have been banned in the US due to life-threatening side effects.

Safe travels!

CHAPTER 6

OTHER USES OF ANTIBIOTICS

Antibiotics for Chronic Inflammation

Some men suffer from inflammation of the prostate gland that is not due to an infection. Having been treated for a presumed infection one or more times, despite no bacteria showing on testing, these men have ongoing inflammation that antibiotics might help with because some antibiotics appear to have anti-inflammatory effects totally aside from their ability to interrupt bacterial growth. Patients with chronic non-bacterial prostatitis are sometimes kept on a low dose of daily antibiotics long term.

Rosacea is inflammation of the facial skin not due to bacterial infection. Topical antibiotics have anti-inflammatory effects, usually in the form of minocycline or erythromycin liquid to the affected area.

Other conditions of chronic inflammation might be due to low-level bacterial infections. These include chronic fatigue, fibromyalgia, Lyme's disease, sarcoidosis, lupus, and rheumatoid arthritis. One theory is that some bacterial strains infiltrate the body's cells, and once inside our cells, they limit the ability of the immune system to find and eliminate the bacteria. This theory gives rise to a number of treatment protocols, including using a combination of pulsed antibiotics, which is on/off treatment schedules with more than one antibiotic. On the other hand, at least part of what causes fibromyalgia symptoms might be abnormal functioning of the energy producing mitochondria. In that case, antibiotic classes that damage mitochondria should be avoided.

The inner machinery that produces cell energy, mitochondria, are probably evolved from bacteria ingested by human cells millions of years ago. Eventually, they were put to work producing internal energy for the human cell, and mitochondria became incorporated into normal cellular function. Therefore, human mitochondria are very similar in structure to free-living bacteria. A common side effect of certain antibiotics is the damaging of mitochondria in normal cells—contributing to antibiotic-associated colitis, for instance.

Antibiotics that target mitochondria include the erythromycins, the tetracyclines, and chloramphenicol.

Antibiotics might limit brain damage by subduing inflammation after a stroke. Animal studies have shown that erythromycin or tetracycline decrease inflammation when given immediately after a stroke. [1] Long-term minocycline (a type of tetracycline) has been shown to help with healing animal versions of human neurological diseases. For example, studies in a small number of humans have demonstrated that treatment with minocycline resulted in fewer relapses of multiple sclerosis. [2] Similarly, long-term minocycline treatment resulted in stabilization and decreased psychiatric symptoms in Huntington's disease. [3]

Research into using antibiotics to prevent atherosclerosis has given mixed results. In some patients, hardening of the arteries is associated with chronic, low-level infection with the bacteria Chlamydia pneumoniae. This is detected by the persistence of antibodies to chlamydia in the bloodstream. Antibiotic therapy has been studied in these patients for variable durations from a 3-day course to a year-long course. Even though this treatment can eliminate chlamydia infection, it does not consistently improve insufficient blood flow to the legs or reduce the risk of heart attack and stroke. It is probable that a more holistic approach is necessary—that is, instead of attacking one bacterial strain with one antibiotic, it makes more sense to correct the body's ability to eliminate bacteria and control inflammation generally.

A holistic approach to controlling bacteria to reduce blood vessel inflammation was first recommended by Elie Mechnikov, the 1908 Nobel Prize winner in medicine. He proposed that aging was because of the body's immune system being so frequently called into action, that it eventually gets indiscriminately activated. Aging, he thought, is the sum of effects of collateral damage coming from widespread immune system activity. He said that death is the final result of chronic inflammation caused by constantly fighting bacterial infections. Mechnikov saw that the hard artery-clogging material (plaque) was full of inflammation, often containing bacteria and white cells (phagocytes) in various stages of ingesting the bacteria. He supposed the inflammation was due to chronic, low-level bacterial infection.

Mechnikov supposed that a lifetime of being under attack by microbes caused the phagocytes to be constantly active. The persistent action of phagocytes was causing side effects, especially damage to the blood vessels. Mechnikov and his colleagues at the Pasteur Institute found that the bacteria that caused milk to ferment created a weak acid (lactic acid). When people ate yogurt, lactic acid produced by the Acidophilus bacteria caused a die-off of the bad bacteria in the colon. Mechnikov was the world's first promoter of what today are called "probiotics." [4]

Antibiotics for Cancer

The relationship of cancer to antibiotics is two-sided. On the one hand, studies have shown a correlation between frequent antibiotic use and the development of breast cancer, and there is evidence that shows the association also holds true for risk of getting a second (recurrent) breast cancer. [5-7]

On the other hand, some antibiotics kill cancer cells because they interrupt the cell cycle of reproduction. Bleomycin is used to treat lung cancer; the related drug mitomycin is used in bladder cancer; doxorubicin and related antibiotics are used in breast cancer; and dactinomycin is used in rare tumors.

More commonly known and less toxic antibiotics are being researched to measure their anticancer activity. Now take a look at the cells that drive cancer growth, called "cancer stem cells." These cells have overly active mitochondria. When cancers are treated with the antibiotics that target mitochondria, the drugs knock their mitochondria out of action, killing the cancer stem cell. Laboratory studies have shown eight different tumor types of cancer respond to these antibiotics: breast, ductal breast carcinoma in situ, ovarian, prostate, lung, pancreatic, melanoma, and glioblastoma (brain). Antibiotics are also being investigated to treat multiple myeloma and liver cancer. At least one of these antibiotics, doxycycline, has the added benefit of promoting the growth of normal stem cells, meaning it has healing properties even while it is killing cancer stem cells. [8]

Antibiotics in Manufacturing

Food animals are given antibiotics not only to prevent and treat infections, but also to promote growth. Growth-promoting antibiotic use has been common practice in the US since 1950, resulting in the growth of larger animals in a shorter time period.

It has been estimated that the volume of nontherapeutic antibiotics used in livestock is eight times the volume consumed for human disease. [9]

Terramycin, a tetracycline type antibiotic, has been routinely used in American beekeeping since the 1950s to treat and prevent foulbrood, a widespread and destructive bee brood disease caused by bacteria. The antibiotic is not well metabolized by the bees, causing trace amounts to be detected unchanged in their honey. It is well documented that like humans, the use of antibiotics causes bees to develop abnormal strains of antibiotic-resistant gut bacteria. In 2005, the US approved a second foulbrood antibiotic, Fumadil-B, while the European Union (EU) was instituting a "no tolerance" policy—EU beekeepers are required to destroy infected colonies rather than treat. [10]

Antibiotics in Paint

Tetracycline is in use worldwide as a paint additive for ship hulls to kill bacteria that would normally grow on the hull. Hull bacteria create a sticky biofilm to which barnacles like to attach, thus contributing to "fouling"—acting to impede boat speed. Tetracycline from the hull paint is rapidly released into the sea where most degrades, but plants and animals absorb or ingest some. The problem of inadvertently causing widespread tetracycline resistance is "being studied" as its risks are significantly less than the poison it replaced. Before tetracycline, tributyltin (TBT) was the most popular anti-fouling chemical, but is toxic to most animals including snails, fish, sea otters, dolphins, and humans. [11]

Sherwin-Williams is a major distributor of antifouling hull paint, and they recently announced a new paint additive they are hoping to market to hospitals, locker rooms, doctor's offices, and daycares. They promise their new product, Paint Shield, will kill 99% of common hospital bacteria on contact. It contains old ingredients (quaternary ammonium compounds, or 'quats') using a new technology to keep it suspended in paint. Presumably this paint will be on the walls, but it is not clear how much hospital infection is caught from the walls. [12]

A new era of quat-resistant bacteria can be expected. These same quats are the antibacterial ingredient in moist disinfectant wipes, and quat-resistant bacteria are found in homes routinely cleaned with antibacterial products. These bacteria are also resistant to a number of other important antibiotics. Quats and their breakdown products might also persist in the environment.

Antibiotics in Distilleries

The process of fermenting grain to make ethanol for fuel or beer and spirits frequently involves contamination by unwanted bacteria. Distillers use antibiotics to control bacterial counts and suppress contamination, and trace amounts of the drugs can persist in the final product. These can include virginiamycin, penicillin, and erythromycin. The distilling industry generates tons of leftover "distillers grains," which are then sold to supplement animal feed for farmed fish, pigs, chicken, and beef herds. The problem is that the distilling process concentrates residual antibiotics, resulting in up to three times the levels in leftover grains as was originally added to the liquid ferment. This can be yet another factor contributing to antibiotic resistance in food animals and in the people who consume them. [13]

Antibiotics in Household Objects

Antibiotics in one form or another are now being incorporated into children's toys, countertops, detergents, sponges, cosmetics, toothpaste, textiles, combs, and brushes. Most of what is used in or on objects is triclosan—in high concentration, it kills bacteria, and in lower concentration, just suppresses bacterial growth. Like any other antibiotic, triclosan promotes drug resistance. Bacteria exposed to low concentrations of triclosan could activate resistance genes that could transfer to other bacteria. Triclosan contributes to the selection of more resistant bacteria, and resistance to triclosan could lead to resistance to other antibiotics. [14]

CHAPTER 7

PENICILLINS

Penicillin was not the first antibiotic, but the first one to be cheaply mass-produced that was effective against a broad spectrum of bacteria. It was also relatively well tolerated, so it was a welcome change from the drugs that came before it, which were based on sulfa, mercury, or arsenic.

The Scottish-born physician Alexander Fleming grew cultures of bacteria in his research lab. In 1928, he happened to leave a culture plate out while away on a month-long vacation. When he returned, he found the neglected bacterial culture had grown moldy. Curiously, the areas around the blooms of mold were clear of any bacteria. The mold was a separate organism, eventually identified as Penicillium notatum. Thus, Fleming accidentally discovered that Penicillium mold kills bacteria. [1]

In fact, molds had been used against infections for years in Chinese medicine and in English folk remedies, but it was Fleming who pushed for his discovery to be purified so that it could be produced as a drug.

There were signs of antibiotic resistance very soon after it was put into use in 1938. As early as 1940, it was detected that some bacteria were capable of producing an enzyme that inactivated penicillin. By 1945, some people were infected with bacteria that were totally resistant to penicillin. That was the same year Fleming shared the Nobel Prize in Medicine with Sir Howard Florey and Ernst Chain for their discovery of the mode of action of penicillin and a method of mass-producing the drug.

All penicillin-related antibiotics have the same basic adverse drug effects, the most significant of which is allergic reaction. The incidence is estimated to be less than 1% to up to 10%, depending on the population studied and the reliability of reports. Allergy can be immediate or may not occur until the second dose is given. It usually takes the form of an itchy rash or welt-like hives.

Rarely, a very severe and sometimes deadly form of allergic reaction can occur, called anaphylaxis: the skin might break out in hives; the throat and tongue swell, blocking the airway; and the circulation collapses, bringing on a state of shock. In most cases, anaphylactic shock can be rapidly reversed with an emergency shot of adrenaline followed by steroids. Anaphylaxis is more frequent in people who have a history of allergies in general, or have asthma.

Other kinds of rashes from penicillin can include sores on the palms, soles, and back of the hands, or red pimples filled with pus. Rarely, a person can get a potential deadly outbreak after taking penicillin, with a painful reddish-purple rash that spreads and blisters, eventually causing the top layer of skin to die and shed. Rarely, penicillin can cause an immune reaction that attacks the small blood vessels. [2]

Amoxicillin is a type of penicillin drug that is better absorbed and stays in the body slightly longer. Amoxicillin and penicillin are equally effective for treatment of tooth abscess, Strep throat, tonsillitis, and some kinds of pneumonia. The side effects are the same, so they will be reviewed together here.

Penicillin or amoxicillin can cause watery and/or bloody stools, with or without stomach cramps and fever. This can happen even as late as two or more months after having taken the last dose. Some cases of especially severe diarrhea are due to the fact that the penicillin killed off beneficial bacteria in the gut. This allows overgrowth of diarrhea-producing bacteria called Clostridium difficile (C diff). Treatment of C diff, in turn, requires more powerful antibiotics. The C diff bacteria produce toxins that severely inflame the large bowel. In extreme cases, C diff diarrhea has to be treated with surgical removal of the entire colon in order to save the patient's life. The change in the bacterial composition of the gut can cause depletions of B2, B9, B12, biotin, and vitamin K. [3]

A related unwanted effect of penicillin is the overgrowth of yeast (*Candida albicans*). This, too, occurs because the antibiotic kills off favorable gut bacteria that was suppressing the growth of too much yeast. After penicillin is taken, the *Candida* yeast is allowed to proliferate unchecked. Yeast overgrowth can cause inflammation and painful sores in the mouth, throat, anus, and vagina. It can also affect the skin, nails, and tongue. Penicillin treatment can cause an overgrowth of bacteria and yeast in the mouth, giving a black, hairy-looking tongue, which is usually accompanied by especially foul breath.

Penicillin commonly causes nausea (and sometimes vomiting), stomach discomfort, and gas. It can cause headache, skin swelling, arthritis, joint pain, muscle pain, and fever. Tooth discoloration (brown, yellow, or gray staining) has been rarely reported, mostly in children.

Rarely, penicillin can cause agitation, anxiety, behavioral changes, confusion, seizures, dizziness, insomnia, and hyperactivity. The patient and family should be aware of these potential drug effects so that the person is not mistakenly labeled as mentally ill.

Penicillin can cause liver dysfunction (including hepatitis with yellow skin and eyes and abnormal liver tests). In high doses given through an intravenous infusion, penicillin can cause abnormal blood counts in red cells, white cells, and platelets, leading to excessive bleeding, especially in patients also on a blood thinner. High doses of penicillin are more likely than lower doses to cause kidney inflammation and nerve damage.

Some resistant bacteria produce enzymes, the penicillinases, which inactivate penicillin. In order to combat this, drug makers have combined amoxicillin with a chemical (clavulanate) that in turn tricks penicillinase into binding with it instead of with the penicillin. While clavulanate is busy neutralizing all of the penicillinase, the penicillin is free to go to work killing the bacteria.

Augmentin or Timentin (amoxicillin with clavulanate) and generic equivalents have all of the potential adverse effects of penicillin and additionally can cause liver damage and gall bladder problems, which are more common with the combo than with amoxicillin alone. Augmentin can interfere with birth control pills, so alternate birth control should be used while on this drug. [4]

Unfortunately, Augmentin is almost always prescribed without first finding out if it is really needed. It is usually given for infections with bacteria that might not even be making the penicillin-blocking enzyme. In these cases, it pushes the bacteria to adapt: they mutate to the point where they can overcome even the clavulanate.

Another way to enhance penicillin is to combine it with another antibiotic. Unasyn is an example of ampicillin combined with the related drug sulbactam. [5] All by itself, sulbactam is not very effective, but when combined with amoxicillin, it partially inhibits penicillinase. This allows the amoxicillin portion to be more effective. Another combo of this type is Zosyn (piperacillin with tazobactam). [6]

There is one use of penicillin that absolutely requires a full 10-day course. When penicillin is given to treat Strep throat infection, it is recommended to take the entire prescription so as to prevent Strep-associated heart valve damage or kidney damage.

CHAPTER 8

CEPHALOSPORINS

Although penicillin originated from a moldy plate, the cephalosporin antibiotics trumped that by coming right out of the sewer. In 1948, Italian researcher Giuseppe Brotzu noticed that some of the common bacterial diseases of the day were rare among inhabitants of Cagliari on the island of Sardinia. The city's sewage emptied into the bay at the Su Siccu port. Despite the fact that the populous swam there and ate raw shellfish from Su Siccu, there were almost none of the water-borne diseases seen elsewhere in Italy, especially cholera and typhoid. [1]

Brotzu suspected the presence of a substance in the polluted water was inhibiting bacteria. He regularly collected sewage samples at the discharge outlets in the bay, and painstakingly coaxed the muck to grow in his laboratory. When he grew cultures of a particular fungus, he found that it produced something that killed off bacteria and named it cephalosporin. Brotzu experimented by injecting it into sick patients with some success. It was later purified in England, and then went into mass production in the US in the mid-1960s.

Cephalosporin antibiotics overlap with penicillin in a portion of their chemical structure, and both classes of antibiotic attack the bacterial cell wall. This kills the bacteria, so they are called bactericidal. Cephalosporins are effective against some bacteria that penicillin leaves alone. [2] Cephalosporins account for the largest share (25%) of the $50 billion global antibiotic market. Since they are used so frequently, they are also major drivers of global antibiotic resistance. [3]

Cephalosporins are classified by generation according to their order of development. The original drugs are called first-generation, and include such familiar names as Duricef, Ancef, and Keflex. They are used to treat uncomplicated skin and soft-tissue infections, uncomplicated urinary tract infections, Strep throat, and are given during surgery to prevent infection.

First-generation cephalosporins, in general, have fewer side effects than penicillin. However, due to the similarity in chemical shapes of these drugs, up to 10% of people allergic to penicillin will also have an allergic reaction if they are given first-generation cephalosporins. In fact, when a couple of employees working in the cephalosporin factory at a US pharma company came down with allergic reactions, they were each found to be allergic to penicillin. These individuals had never taken cephalosporins, but industrial exposure was enough to provoke cross-allergic reactions. Another liability of the similarity to penicillin is the tendency for bacteria to become resistant to the cell wall-destroying activity.

First-Generation Cephalosporins (* taken by mouth)

cefadroxil (Duricef)*	cefazedone
cephradine (Velocef, Intracef)*	cefazolin (Ancef, Kefazol)
cephalexin (Keflex, Keftabs)*	cephalothin (Keflin)
cephaloridine (Ceporin)	cephapirin

Duricef, Keflex, and Velocef have identical potential adverse drug effects. Manufacturers advise that these drugs are unlikely to be beneficial if they are prescribed "just in case" there is a bacterial infection and should not be used for symptoms of a virus infection. They also should not be given preventively, unless the person is undergoing surgery.

These drug labels carry a prominent warning about the possibility of allergic reactions. A drug rash can rapidly progress to tongue swelling with trouble breathing. Allergy is more likely if the person has a known penicillin allergy. If that is the case, the doctor can give the first dose in the office or emergency room, and observe for any reaction since over 90% of people with penicillin allergies are likely to be fine on cephalosporins.

Cephalosporins can cause nausea, vomiting, and stomach pain. Antibiotic-associated diarrhea from overgrowth of C difficile may be watery and bloody. It may resolve when the antibiotic is stopped, but some cases could require intensive treatment with yet another antibiotic. There are some strains of C difficile that produce toxic substances, leading to such severe colitis that surgery is necessary. Diarrhea can also be delayed and might show up two months after the last dose of cephalosporin. These drugs should be used with extreme caution in people who already have a colon condition.

Another effect of cephalosporin's suppression of normal bacteria is the overgrowth of yeast. *Candida* infections of the mouth (thrush) or vagina (vaginal yeast infection) may require anti-fungal treatment.

The body eliminates the first-generation cephalosporin drugs through the kidneys. Anyone with kidney disease should be given a lesser dose, and these individuals should have kidney tests while on the antibiotic. Increased liver enzymes, abnormal blood cell counts, and rashes can occur. First – and second-generation cephalosporins can cause the body to make antibodies against its own red blood cells; rarely this can progress rapidly to severe anemia. [4,5]

The safety of these drugs has not been adequately studied in pregnancy or in nursing mothers. Some cephalosporins can trigger seizures, especially in people with kidney disease. In addition to any of the above effects, Ancef can cause a positive test for sugar in the urine.

The best way to decide on appropriate antibiotic treatment is to get a sample from the infected body part, and culture it in a growth medium in the lab. Whatever grows is tested against several antibiotics. One study showed that when Keflex (cephalexin) was given in the absence of the results of bacteriologic testing, it failed to eradicate deep skin infections about a quarter of the time. [6]

Some doctors wonder if any antibiotics are necessary for skin abscesses (boils). One study looked at the clearance of infection after abscesses were drained: infection cleared on its own in 90% of patients who were not given any antibiotic, while with cephalexin treatment infection cleared only 84% of the time. [7]

In a 2005 study, it was reported that once a day cefadroxil (Duricef) treatment of Strep throat failed to eradicate infection nearly 20% of the time. Even more drug resistance is likely to have occurred in the past decade since that report was created. [8]

Second-generation cephalosporins are used to treat infections of the sinuses, the nose and throat, airways and lungs, middle ear infections, sore throat and tonsillitis, bronchitis, and uncomplicated urinary tract infections. They can be used for more complicated infections of the skin and soft tissues, and are used against abdominal and gynecologic infections.

Second-Generation Cephalosporins (* taken by mouth)

cefaclor (Ceclor, Raniclor)*	cefamandole (Mandol)
cefuroxime (Ceftin, Zinacef)*	cefmetazole (Zefazone)
cefprozil (Cefzil)*	cefotetan (Cefotan)
loracarbef (Lorabid)*	cefoxitin (Mefoxin)

Each generation of cephalosporins consist of modified drug molecules, with the idea of making them more difficult to be recognized by bacteria. Unfortunately, many types of bacteria have already outwitted the altered chemical structure of the second-generation drugs, and antibiotic resistance is not uncommon.

Like the first-generation cephalosporins, Ceclor and Ceftin can cause diarrhea, nausea, and vomiting; overgrowth of yeast; and C difficile associated colitis. They can interfere with tests for sugar, cause elevated liver enzymes, and cause the body to make antibodies that attack red blood cells. [9]

Ceftin and Ceclor can cause an excess of allergic cells in the blood (eosinophilia). Ceftin can cause loss of appetite, headache, chest pain, shortness of breath, chills, tiredness, and thirst. Ceclor can cause an allergic response called serum sickness, characterized by joint pains, rash, and sometimes fever. Ceclor can damage the kidneys. Rarely, psychiatric symptoms have been reported with Ceclor, such as hyperactivity, agitation, nervousness, insomnia, confusion, stiff muscles, dizziness, hallucinations, and sleepiness. [10]

Two decades ago, there was a 94% success rate when middle ear infections in children were treated with cefaclor (Ceclor). [11] This figure has stayed relatively steady, with a 2005 study showing about the same. [12] Cefuroxime (Ceclor) is reported to be about 93% effective in treating adults with recurrent bronchitis when that bronchitis has been proven to be bacterial (most bronchitis is viral). [13]

The third-generation cephalosporins are strongly bactericidal when used for abdominal infections, pneumonia, and other serious infections. Unlike the earlier generations, third-generation cephalosporins penetrate the protective barrier surrounding the brain and spinal cord. Thus they are used for bacterial meningitis (infection of the brain lining). Bacteria will rapidly become resistant to third-generation cephalosporins unless the patient is simultaneously treated with another antibiotic from a different class.

Third-Generation Cephalosporins (*taken by mouth)

cefdinir (Omnicef)*	cefditoren (Spectracef)*
cefixime (Suprax)*	cefpodoxime (Vantin)*
ceftibuten (Cedax)*	cefsulodin (Takesulin)
cefcapene (Flomox)	ceftizoxime (Cefizox)
cefetamet (Altamet)	ceftriaxone (Rocephin)
cefmenoxime (Bestcall, Bestron)	latamoxef (or moxalactam)
cefoperazone (Cefobid)	(Shiomarin), is an oxacephem
cefotaxime (Claforan)	flomoxef (Flumarin), is an oxacephem
cefpiramide	

Two additional third-generation drugs, ceftazidime (Fortaz, Tazicef, Tazidime) and cefoperazone (Cefobid), are given intravenously for treatment of infections from the bacteria Pseudomonas. These bacteria can cause life-threatening illness in people who have weak immune systems, such as premature babies, people with AIDS, and cancer chemotherapy patients. In fact, Pseudomonas can be so deadly that it is being investigated as a biological warfare agent. [14]

The third-generation drugs can cause any of the same adverse effects of the earlier generation drugs, including various symptoms and abnormal lab tests. The manufacturer of generic Suprax reports that 30% of adult patients get some sort of digestive side effects, including heartburn, nausea, vomiting, excess gas, pain, and diarrhea. Overgrowth of yeast, infection with resistant superbugs, and C difficile colitis are possible. The third-generation drugs are passed through the liver as well as the kidneys, and there are rare reports of liver damage while on these drugs. [15]

The pharmaceutical company's cefixime (Suprax) package insert reports failure rates of 18% to 31% when it is used to treat middle ear infections in children. [15] A 2013 study found a 7% failure rate when cefixime (Suprax) was used for treatment of gonorrhea. [16] The package insert for cefdinir (Omnicef) describes failure rates up to 20% when given for pneumonia, and failure rates of about 10% when given for Strep throat. [17]

The fourth (and subsequent) generations of cephalosporins are sometimes called gorilla-cillins, mocking the ever-increasing need to come up with stronger medicines to overcome drug resistance. Examples include cefepime (Maxipime) and cefpirome (Cefrom). These drugs are exclusively used for infections with superbugs as seen in hospitalized patients. They are always given along with antibiotics of another class.

Like all antibiotics disturbing the normal gut bacterial balance, cephalosporins can cause depletions of B2, B9, B12, biotin, and vitamin K. [18]

CHAPTER 9

TETRACYCLINES

Tetracyclines were discovered in the late 1940s. The first tetracyclines were naturally made by a couple different strains of bacteria that lived in the soil. It is presumed the tetracycline-producing bacteria were poisoning competing bacteria of a different species. In just a few years, chemists figured out how to modify the tetracycline molecule in the lab to make related drugs, and today all drugs in this class are semi-synthetic.

It is possible that the discovery in the modern era was really a re-discovery. Tetracycline has a tendency to lodge in the bones, and anthropologists have discovered tetracycline in Nubian skeletons from around 350 AD. The Nubian civilization along the Nile River (in what is now lower Egypt/ upper Sudan) cultivated a grain-based alcoholic beverage, something like beer. The initial explanation for the antibiotics in their bones was that perhaps their beer was made from grains that were contaminated with tetracycline-making bacteria.

That theory was modified when some of the skeletons were found to be saturated with tetracycline, including those of a 4-year-old child. It is unlikely that much tetracycline would be from contamination, and instead it looks like these people had been intentionally treated. [1]

Common tetracyclines and example brand names:

tetracycline

doxycycline (Doryx)

lymecycline (Tetralysal)

meclocycline (Meclan)

chlortetracycline (Aureomycin)   methacycline (Rondomycin)
oxytetracycline (Terramycin)   minocycline (Minocin)
demeclocycline (Declomycin)   rolitetracycline

Tetracyclines work by inhibiting the ability of bacteria to make protein. They can be used to treat respiratory infections, intestinal infections, urinary infections, and sexually transmitted diseases (especially syphilis and chlamydia). The most common uses of tetracyclines in America are for treatment of the skin conditions acne and rosacea. Tetracyclines can be applied directly on the skin or taken internally.

Tetracycline is also used to prevent and treat malaria, which is caused by parasites rather than bacteria. Tetracyclines are the go-to drugs for treating proven cases of anthrax, the plague, Rocky Mountain spotted fever, Lyme disease, and Legionnaire's disease. Tetracycline is often effective against Staph bacteria that have developed resistance to penicillin. Some of the tetracyclines have anti-viral activity. [2]

Tetracyclines have several actions that go well beyond treating bacterial infections. They seem to quiet down inflammation, and this may be a major reason they help with rosacea and acne. [3] These drugs are being investigated to treat rheumatoid arthritis. Doxycycline also treats inflammatory eye conditions such as corneal ulcers. There is promising research into the ability of tetracycline drugs to limit brain damage after a stroke, and researchers are exploring the possibility of using tetracyclines to slow progression of dementia in Alzheimer's disease, Huntington's disease, and Parkinson's disease. [4] Doxycycline has been shown to decrease the development of diabetes in diabetic-prone rats. In people, low dose daily doxycycline slows the progression of the eye disease retinopathy, which is a leading cause of blindness in diabetics. Tetracyclines have been demonstrated to suppress the growth and to kill cancer cells in experimental models of prostate tumors, breast cancer, leukemia, osteosarcoma, and mesothelioma. [5]

Tetracyclines, like all antibiotics that treat a broad spectrum of bacteria, can cause an imbalance in the normal gut bacteria and resultant overgrowth of yeast, vaginal yeast infections, as well as C difficile associated colitis with profuse watery, bloody diarrhea. Antibiotics cause depletions of vitamins B2 (riboflavin), B9 (folate), B12 (cobalamin), biotin, and vitamin K. [6]

Tetracyclines have some unique potential adverse effects too. They cause extreme sun sensitivity (photosensitivity), increasing the risk of sunburn. The drug should be stopped at the first sign of skin redness. Tetracyclines cause yellow, gray, or brownish discoloration of teeth, especially in the fetus or young child, although grayish tooth discoloration can happen in adults. Tetracycline can delay bone growth in children. Rarely, tetracyclines can cause a buildup of fluid pressure in the brain, causing severe headaches and vision problems. [7]

There are two general groups of tetracyclines. Those that are water-soluble are excreted through the kidneys and can cause kidney failure in people who already have kidney problems. Those that are fat-soluble (oily) are metabolized through the liver, where they can cause fatty deposits in the liver and liver failure. Liver injury is more likely when expired lots of tetracyclines are consumed.

Tetracycline adverse effects:

allergic reaction	itching
loss of appetite	dark-colored urine
sore mouth	light-colored bowel movements
upset stomach	extreme tiredness or weakness
stomach pain	confusion
vomiting	joint stiffness or swelling
diarrhea	unusual bleeding or bruising
itching of the rectum or vagina	decreased urination
extreme photosensitivity, sunburn	throat sores
changes in skin color	fever or chills
severe headache	fatty liver
blurred vision	liver failure
skin rash	kidney failure
hives	decreased bone growth
difficulty breathing or swallowing	worsening of systemic lupus erythromatosis

yellowing of the skin or eyes	worsening of myasthenia gravis
low white blood cell count	anemia
low platelet count	effects on fetus: discolored teeth, inguinal hernia
increased brain pressure	

The instructions for taking tetracycline antibiotics should be followed precisely. The water soluble, short-acting drugs (plain tetracycline, chlortetracycline, oxytetracycline, demeclocycline, and methacycline) should be taken with a full glass of water, either two hours after eating or two hours before eating. Doxycycline and minocycline can be taken with food, but not with antacids, iron supplements, or calcium supplements. There have been rare instances of ulceration of the esophagus from taking a tetracycline capsule with minimal water just before bed.

Many bacteria have adapted to get around the action of tetracycline. Some resistant bacteria have made enzymes (chemicals) to inactivate tetracycline. Two other mechanisms account for most of the tetracycline resistance: a pump that shunts tetracycline out of the bacterial cell and the ability to block the attachment of tetracycline.

Tetracycline is widely used in animal food production. Chicken feed is commonly heavily dosed with tetracycline. Public demand for antibiotic-free chicken has recently led major chicken breeders to begin phasing out intensive antibiotic use in some of their production lines. This is possible by making the pens less crowded, cleaning the pens more frequently, providing better ventilation, and increasing the use of vaccines. Pig and beef production continue to use tetracycline and other antibiotics, contributing to global antibiotic resistance. A high percentage of workers from swine slaughterhouses have tetracycline-resistant bacteria growing on their skin. [8]

CHAPTER 10

MACROLIDES (ERYTHROMYCIN AND RELATED DRUGS)

The macrolide family of antibiotics includes erythromycin (E-Mycine, EES, ERYC), clarithromycin (Biaxin), and azithromycin (Zithromax); a related drug is telithromycin (Ketek). Dirithromycin (Dynabac) and roxithromycin (Rulid, Surlid) are macrolides not sold in the US.

Erythromycin is a natural chemical made by bacteria found in the soil. It was first isolated in 1949 by a researcher at Eli Lilly, an American global pharmaceutical company, who was working on soil samples collected by Abelardo Aguilar, a Lilly medical doctor in the Philippines. This was a discovery of worldwide importance at the time, because many infections were starting to show penicillin resistance. Macrolides are an alternative for people with penicillin or cephalosporin allergies. Aguilar never received any compensation beyond his usual salary for his contribution, although he formally asked for a $500 million share of Lilly's immense profits from sales of erythromycin. He eventually resigned from the company and returned to providing medical services to the poor. [1]

All antibiotic package inserts lead with strong advice to the physician that prescribing in the absence of a proven or strongly suspected bacterial infection, or giving antibiotics only for prevention, is unlikely to provide benefit to the patient while increasing the risk of drug resistance. Indeed, some bacteria showed erythromycin resistance as early as 1955. Resistance can occur when bacteria change the shape of their protein-making site where macrolides act or develop a mechanism to pump the antibiotic out of the bacterial cell.

In the 1980s, two new drugs were developed by chemically altering the natural erythromycin molecule. These are called "semi-synthetic" and were designed with the hopes of bypassing erythromycin resistance. Clarithromycin (Biaxin) was developed at Taisho Pharmaceuticals in Japan, and azithromycin (Zithromax) at Pliva Pharmaceuticals in Croatia. [2]

The macrolides act by inhibiting the ability of bacteria to make proteins. They suppress the growth of bacteria at medium doses and kill bacteria at higher doses. A huge advantage is that these drugs are concentrated in the tissues and cells more than in the blood. For example, Biaxin concentration in tonsils is twice as high and in lungs over four times as high as in the blood. This keeps the chance of system-wide side effects at a minimum while the drug is concentrating in the sick tissues where it is really needed.

Macrolides also modulate immune responses. The drugs show a preference for infection-fighting white blood cells, which in turn go directly to the site of infection and seek out bacteria. One study of azithromycin (Zithromax) showed it makes the immune response more vigorous at first, then decreases inflammation over the long run. Macrolides have some ability to decrease the tendency of the airways to constrict, limit the flow of mucous, and reduce the ability of bacteria to stick to the airway passages. Macrolides are sometimes given as anti-inflammatories in low doses for a lifetime in chronic lung diseases such as cystic fibrosis or asthma. [3]

Macrolides can treat anything penicillin is used for, such as bronchitis, pneumonia, skin infections, gonorrhea, chlamydia, pelvic inflammatory disease, and tuberculosis in AIDS patients. They treat atypical community acquired pneumonia, sometimes called "walking pneumonia," and are given with a second antibiotic plus an acid suppressing medication to treat the ulcer-causing H pylori infection.

All of the macrolides carry warnings about possible interference with transmission of electrical impulses in the heart and the possibility of causing irregular heartbeats, which can be fatal. The risk of heart problems from macrolides is higher if the patient already has heart rhythm problems; is also taking certain heart medications, psychiatric drugs, or quinolone antibiotics; or has insufficient potassium, calcium, or magnesium.

Macrolides carry warnings about the potential to cause liver injury, ranging from elevated liver blood tests with no symptoms to fatal liver failure. Like any other antibiotic, these drugs can upset the balance of normal gut microorganisms, causing an overgrowth of yeast or C difficile colitis with watery, bloody diarrhea.

The most common adverse effects are gastrointestinal: nausea, stomach cramping, pain, constipation, or diarrhea are common. Vomiting and inflammation of the pancreas are less common. A person may be allergic to macrolides and experience a swollen tongue, constricting throat, and welt-like rash. Macrolides can cause a number of lab abnormalities, including elevated liver enzymes, low blood sugar, decreased white blood cell count, and elevated kidney tests. They cause depletion of vitamins B2 (riboflavin), B9 (folate), B12 (cobalamin), biotin, and vitamin K.

Macrolides can cause a worsening of the neurologic disorder myasthenia gravis and might also cause new onset of myasthenia. Symptoms include drooping eyelids, trouble swallowing, and weakness when getting out of a chair or trying to lift arms overhead.

In addition, there have been reports of macrolide drugs causing:

painful inflammation of tongue	hallucinations
discoloration of tongue and teeth	insomnia
anemia	depression
low platelet count	manic behavior
hearing loss, ringing in ears	nightmares
dizziness	psychosis
sense of smell loss	tremor
taste perversion or loss	low blood pressure

kidney injury

anxiety

behavioral changes

aggressiveness

confusion

convulsions

depersonalization

disorientation

palpitations

fatigue

heartburn

joint pain

black outs

rash

swelling

The macrolides strongly inhibit a liver enzyme responsible for metabolizing certain drugs. When a person taking daily medication then takes any of the macrolides in addition, the liver might not break down the daily drugs as efficiently, making the patient more likely to experience drug side effects. Macrolides should not be taken with antacids or ergot-type drugs (derived from ergot fungi group), such as some medications taken for migraine headaches.

Drugs with possible interactions with macrolides:

amlodipine (Norvasc)

diltiazem (Cardizem, Tiazac)

nicardipine (Cardene SR)

nifedipine (Procardia)

nisoldipine (Sular)

verapamil (Calan, Verelan, Covera-HS)

amiodarone

methadone

lithium

amitriptyline (Elavil)

citalopram (Celexa)

blood thinners

simvastatin (Vytorin)

atorvastatin (Lipitor)

digoxin

midazolam (Versed)

triazolam (Halcion)

carbamazepine (Tegretol)

cimetidine (Tagamet)

clozapine (Clozaril)

colchicine

theophylline

ranitidine bismuth (Zantac)

tolterodine (Detrol)

sildenafil (Viagra)

antacids

ergot drugs

zidovudine, ritonavir and other anti-viral drugs

rifampicin and related anti-TB drugs

alprazolam(Xanax)

Erythromycin and Zithromax are assigned the FDA pregnancy category

B. The B rating either means animal studies don't show a risk but human studies are lacking or can mean animal studies have shown an adverse effect but human studies have not. This uncertainty limits their use in pregnant women. The drugs do pass into breast milk. Biaxin is assigned pregnancy category C, meaning animal studies have shown a risk to the offspring but there are not sufficient studies in humans. Animal studies also show Biaxin passes into breast milk.

Drug studies cited by the manufacturer on the package inserts of the macrolides report anywhere from 71% to 100% effectiveness in eradicating infection, depending on the bacteria and the setting, or up to a 30% failure rate. [4,5,6]

A drug with a related chemical structure is telithromycin (Ketek). Ketek was approved by the FDA in 2004 based on very shaky evidence of safety and effectiveness. On its first review, the FDA did not approve the drug because of concerns for liver injury and vision problems. The manufacturer, Sanofi-Aventis, funded a study and recruited 1,800 physicians, paying them $400 per patient enrolled to take the drug. The doctor who recruited the most patients was investigated by the FDA, and they found she had falsified medical records and completely fabricated the paperwork of fictional enrollees. This led to a 57-month prison sentence on a federal conviction of fraud. Three other doctors' offices were referred for criminal investigation, but that is only less than 1% of the doctors financially incentivized to prescribe a drug that the FDA bothered to investigate.

Nevertheless, the study results were presented for review to a drug-approving panel who had no knowledge of the criminal discoveries being uncovered by FDA staffers. The panel voted 11 to 1 to approve Ketek solely on the basis that it was *at least as good as existing drugs*. Seven months after it was on the market in the US, a patient who had been prescribed Ketek for a mild upper respiratory infection died from liver failure. Soon there were two other liver failure cases reported by the same medical center. By June of 2006, there were 23 cases of severe liver injury and 12 cases of liver failure—4 of them fatal, all linked to Ketek. Eventually, the FDA called for stronger label warnings about the possibility of liver failure and limited the use of Ketek only to treatment of community-acquired pneumonia. [7]

In addition to all of the adverse effects of the macrolides, the Ketek package insert carries a Black Box Warning about the possibility of causing or worsening myasthenia gravis. Ketek uniquely can cause vision problems including blurred vision and trouble focusing. There have been reports of losing consciousness, prompting a bold font warning against operating machinery. [8]

In addition to the drugs listed above for macrolides, Ketek could have drug interactions with the following:

itraconazole (Sporanox)	metoprolol (Lopressor)
ketoconazole (Nizoral)	digoxin
grapefruit juice	theophylline
simvastatin (Zocor)	oral contraceptivesrifampin
midazolam (Versed)	paroxetine (Paxil)

The macrolide antibiotics can be lifesaving in certain conditions and may prolong the life of a child with cystic fibrosis or prevent tuberculosis in an AIDS patient. However, for mild to moderate infections in the usually well population, it is imperative to heed the warning against taking these drugs unless infection with bacteria is proven or strongly suspected. Even when bacteria are responsible, a course of antibiotics may not be the best thing. A study reported in the *Journal of the American Medical Association* reported that neither antibiotics nor nasal steroid sprays were effective for treating sinusitis. [9] In cases of pneumonia in persons who are not sick enough to be hospitalized, it is estimated that less than 50% are due to bacteria, yet it is common for 100% of such patients to be prescribed antibiotics. [10] The cost of obtaining sputum samples or nasal swabs to send for culture is worth it to avoid the human cost if we don't prevent drug side effects and antibiotic resistance.

CHAPTER 11

AMINOGLYCOSIDES

Aminoglycosides are a group of chemicals made by a particular type of soil bacteria, *Streptomyces griseus*. In 1943, the first aminoglycoside, streptomycin, was isolated and named by graduate student Albert Schatz while working in a lab at Rutgers University. It was the first antibiotic derived from bacteria and the first cure for tuberculosis (TB). Along with TB, streptomycin treats the plague, cholera, typhoid, and other serious, life-threatening infections such as heart valve infections and war wounds. In addition to being effective against bacteria, aminoglycosides treat some fungal infections. Like most other antibiotics, aminoglycosides are not effective against influenza, the common cold, or other viral infections. [1]

Discoverer Schatz was convinced by his lab director, Selman Waksman, to sign off on any patent rights in an effort to make the drug cheaply available to as many people as possible. Schatz sued when he found Waksman had arranged to get 20% of the royalties; the legal action led to recognition of Schatz as "co-discoverer" and allowed him 3% royalties. [2] Two years later, both men were nominated for the Nobel Prize in medicine, but Waksman alone won the award. Although Waksman is listed on the Nobel organization website as getting the award for the discovery of streptomycin, the actual prize presentation had been carefully reworded in consideration of the known facts; it says Waksman was awarded the prize for "ingenious, systematic and successful studies of the soil microbes that have led to the discovery of streptomycin." [3]

Waksman didn't mention Schatz at all in his acceptance speech at the awards banquet before the King of Sweden. In his published Nobel lecture, Waksman only mentions Schatz in his closing paragraph, among a list of over 20 other names of "collaborators, associates and students." [4]

Aminoglycoside drugs include:

Amikacin (Amikin)	neomycin (Mycifradin, Myciguent)
Gentamicin (Garamycin, G-Mycin)	netilmicin (Netromycin)
lanomycin	paromomycin
kanamycin (Kantrex)	tobramycin (TOBI, Tobrex, Nebcin)

Aminoglycosides are not absorbed from the stomach; in fact, if they are taken by mouth, 100% of the substance is eliminated in the stool, largely unchanged. Therefore, these drugs are given intravenously and also work externally on the skin or in the eye. They penetrate bacterial cells and inhibit the manufacture of proteins. This kills the bacteria, though the smarter bugs have developed several mechanisms of resistance: altering the site where the drug binds, blocking the drug from entering the cell, and chemically inactivating it.

Aminoglycoside package inserts carry Black Box warnings about being poisonous to the kidneys and ears, and toxic to the neuromuscular system. For this reason, blood tests are checked frequently to guide dosing at the minimum effective levels, but that is not always helpful because kidney damage sometimes occurs after just one dose. When biochemists modified portions of the aminoglycoside molecule responsible for the worst side effects (ear damage and kidney injury), the molecule lost antibiotic properties, preventing modification from reducing those risk factors. Unfortunately, these powerful drugs come with significant risks, so should only be used when there is proven resistance to less toxic alternatives.

They are assigned pregnancy category D, meaning that studies have shown they cause harm to the fetus. Infants, children, elderly, and people who are dehydrated are especially vulnerable to toxicity. Any other drug that affects the kidneys, ears, or nervous system should be avoided while taking aminoglycosides. [5,6]

Intravenous aminoglycoside potential toxicities:

kidney failure	spasm of air passages
deafness	aggravation of Parkinson's disease
ringing in the ears	aggravation of myasthenia gravis
blindness	anemia
delayed electrical transmission in the heart	low white blood cell count
abnormal heart rhythm	low platelets
allergy with potential life threatening swelling	increased liver enzymes
C difficile associated profuse watery, bloody diarrhea	loss of appetite
dizziness	nausea
numbness	vomiting
skin tingling	weight loss
twitching	tongue inflammation
convulsion	increased salivation
seizure	bleeding into the stomach or bowel
brain disease	hair loss
excess fluid in the head	fever
confusion	enlarged spleen
depression	enlarged liver
headache	joint pain
weakness	breathing difficulty
paralysis	low sodium, potassium, calcium, magnesium, iron
weak breathing muscles	depletion of vitamins A, B12, K [7]

Tobramycin is also used in an inhaled form for cystic fibrosis (TOBI inhaler). Some of the antibiotic is absorbed into the system, especially because it is prescribed for extended durations of daily use. The TOBI inhaler label has the same warnings as the intravenous form regarding damage to hearing, kidney injury, and neuromuscular paralysis. [8]

Gentamicin (Genoptic, Garamycin) and tobramycin (Tobrex) are available in topical forms to treat eye conditions and minor skin infections. In these forms, allergic reactions to the drugs are still possible, but they lack serious toxicity to the kidneys, ears, and nervous system. [9]

Some human diseases are caused by faulty genetic codes. For example, in cystic fibrosis, the genetic programming for lung proteins is defective. The coding for muscle protein is abnormal in some forms of muscular dystrophy. On the other hand, aminoglycosides work by interfering with how the bacterial cell reads genetic information to make proteins. Starting with the aminoglycoside backbone, biochemists designed some compounds that would intentionally miss-read very specific portions of the human genetic code. In particular, the drug would skip over only the bit that is genetically abnormal. For example, if a gene spells out the code CATCATXCAT, and that 'X' causes the body to make a faulty lung protein resulting in cystic fibrosis, the designer drug would cause the cell to read it as CATCATCAT, skipping over the X. [10] There are already patents on such novel drugs that target specific genetic diseases. This innovative research takes antibiotic discoveries to the next level of possible benefit for mankind.

CHAPTER 12

SULFA DRUGS

Sulfa drugs were the first broadly effective oral antibiotics. They were discovered by Gerhard Domagk when he was working at the massive chemical industrial complex of IG Farben. Domagk and his team were systematically studying a variety of dye compounds to see if any happened to have antibiotic effect. In the early 1930s, they found a red dye that inhibited bacterial infections in mice. Strangely, this effect was seen only in animals and not in laboratory flasks or culture plates of bacteria. It was presumed that something in the body activated the drug. Domagk and his colleague patented the compound as Prontosil, but did not release it for a couple of years while they conducted more testing.

One of the test subjects was Domagk's own daughter, who had gotten infected from an unsterilized needle. She was cured of infection by Prontosil, but it left her with a reddish tint to her skin. Between a dirty needle and red skin, it must not have been easy being the child of an experimental doctor. Domagk was awarded the Nobel Prize in medicine in 1939 for his discovery, but apprehended by the German police and forced to write a letter to the Nobel committee rejecting the Prize. (The Germans had been upset with the Nobel organization ever since their 1935 award to German peace activist Carl von Ossietzky.) [1]

Incidentally, IG Farben was the single biggest contributor to Adolf Hitler's election campaign and garnered the greatest profits as a war machine. IG Farben directors were tried and found guilty of numerous war crimes in the post war Nuremberg trials, which included details of the company's role at Auschwitz concentration camp. [2]

Other researchers soon discovered that inside the body, Prontosil was split into two parts—one part was the active antibiotic. When this active part was examined, it was found to be a dye that had been around since 1906, its patent long since expired. So the patented Prontosil was useless, since anyone could manufacture the unpatented active drug.

The active ingredient is chemically known as sulfonamide. Several different forms of sulfonamide antibiotics exist today. They are most commonly prescribed in combination with other drugs.

> Trimethoprim-Sulfamethoxazole (Bactrim, Bactrim DS, Septra)
>
> Erythromycin/sulfafurazole (Pediazole)
>
> Trimethoprim (Trimpex, Proloprim, and Primsol)
>
> Co-Trimoxazole (Septrin)

Sulfonamides work by inhibiting bacteria from making folate, a B vitamin essential to bacterial growth and reproduction. The drugs are used to treat adult bronchitis, children's ear infections, traveler's diarrhea, urinary tract infections, and some pneumonia. These drugs should not be used to treat Strep throat and should not be given unless a bacterial infection is strongly suspected or proven and testing shows the bacteria is sensitive to sulfonamides. Overuse can promote the development of resistant bacteria.

Allergy and other hypersensitivity reactions are the most common adverse effects of sulfonamides and combination drugs. Reactions can be as mild as an itchy rash or as severe as throat swelling and death from rapid lung congestion causing inability to breathe. In higher doses, these drugs can cause extreme immune reactions causing a life-threatening total body rash that can progress to the skin sloughing off. [3,4]

The drug package inserts on all sulfonamide-containing antibiotics carry Black Box warnings about potentially fatal allergic and immune reactions. The drug should be stopped at the first sign of a rash or bruising, or a new onset of cough, fever, or joint pain. These drugs can cause sudden liver toxicity with rapid death of liver cells, thus should be stopped if there is any sign of yellowing skin. The sulfonamides can cause sudden severe anemia, low blood count, and other blood abnormalities. They should be stopped at any sign of paleness or weakness. Like all antibiotics, the sulfonamides can cause C difficile associated colitis with profuse watery, bloody diarrhea.

Potential adverse effects of sulfonamides:

high potassium	vomiting
low sodium	abdominal pain
depletion of vitamin B2	loss of appetite
depletion of vitamin B9	inflammation of pancreas
depletion of vitamin B12	diarrhea
depletion of vitamin K	yeast infection
rash	light sensitivity
bruising	meningitis
skin sloughing	convulsions
blistering of skin	nerve pain
itching	numbness
fever	difficulty walking
chills	dizziness
joint pain	ringing in the ears
swollen throat and trouble breathing	hearing loss
lung congestion	eye inflammation
shortness of breath	headache
cough	hallucinations
blood vessel inflammation	depression
swelling	apathy
sore throat	nervousness
anemia	muscle pain
low white cell count	insomnia
low platelet count	weakness
yellowing of eyes or skin	fatigue
inflammation of the heart	blood in stool

inflamed tongue	bleeding skin
nausea	blood in urine
low blood sugar	kidney failure

Pediazole is a combination drug with the antibiotics erythromycin and sulfafurazole or sulfisoxazole. It has all of the potential effects listed for sulfonamides, but also the effects of erythromycin (see chapter 10). Bactrim and Septra are brand names for the combination of trimethoprim and sulfamethoxazole. Trimethoprim also blocks the bacteria's use of folate (vitamin B9). [5]

Sulfonamides should not be given to anyone with liver disease, kidney disease, or impaired bone marrow production of red and white blood cells. They should not be used in people with a genetic enzyme deficiency of G6PD or the inherited disorder called porphyria. They should be avoided during pregnancy because it is possible that a fetus could be born with serious birth defects. The incidence of any of these adverse drug effects is especially high in persons with AIDS.

Sulfonamides interfere with many specialty lab tests and can have dangerous interactions with scores of prescription drugs. Tell your doctor and pharmacist of *every* other medication you are on, and read the package insert to double check as well.

Sulfonamides are not the same as sulfites, which are in beer, wine, and food preservatives; or sulfates, which are natural substances formed in the body from metabolizing the protein we eat. Allergy to a sulfonamide antibiotic does not necessarily mean the person is allergic to sulfa. However, there is potential for cross-allergy from related (non-antibiotic) drugs that have a sulfonamide structure, such as some water pills, anti-diabetic drugs, arthritis medications, seizure medications, and drugs for HIV infection.

One notorious brand of sulfonamide was a preparation made by the Massengill pharmaceutical company. A company chemist mixed it into a raspberry-flavored liquid by dissolving it in a solvent called diethylene glycol (DEG). Massengill called their preparation Elixir

Sulfanilamide and marketed it for a wide variety of ailments from sore throat to gonorrhea. The Massengill chemist was not aware of medical reports that had been published describing DEG as a fatal poison. After more than 100 deaths across the country, most of them children, the cause was traced to the Massengill product. In those days, there was no requirement for safety testing or animal testing before marketing, but there was a national uproar and demand for justice. Massengill owner, Dr. Samuel Evans Massengill, said, "My chemists and I deeply regret the fatal results, but there was no error in the manufacture of the product. We have been supplying a legitimate professional demand and not once could have foreseen the unlooked-for results. I do not feel that there was any responsibility on our part." The company also sold preparations of arsenic, mercury, strychnine, methadone, and a cough syrup containing cannabis and chloroform. The Massengill chemist committed suicide while awaiting trial. [6]

The company got away with a fine for mislabeling their drug as an elixir, which means dissolved in alcohol. Despite the tragedy, Massengill remained a successful pharmaceutical firm until merging with Beecham in 1971. The incident was instrumental in passage of the Federal Food, Drug, and Cosmetic Act of 1938, consisting of new laws requiring pharmaceutical firms to conduct safety testing—something taken for granted today.

DEG is used in plastic manufacture as a machine lubricant and in brake fluid. Worldwide, DEG poisoning from drug preparations unrelated to sulfonamides continues it has been found in a teething salve, toothpaste, over the counter sedatives, medical ointment, a diuretic (water pill), cold remedies, a medication for gall bladder problems, pediatric enema fluid, blood vessel disease injections, intravenous pain reliever, and an arthritis medication. Many, but not all of these products, originated in China. [7]

CHAPTER 13

QUINOLONES – THE "FLOXIN" DRUGS

Many of the early antibiotics were discovered in nature, especially by studying the products of mold (as in the discovery of penicillin) or soil and water bacteria (as in discovery of erythromycin, streptomycin, and tetracycline). In contrast, the first quinolone was created entirely in the chemistry lab. In 1962, nalidixic acid was unexpectedly discovered while researchers were attempting to make synthetic chloroquine, an anti-malaria drug. Nalidixic acid was incidentally found to have an inhibiting effect on bacterial growth. By the late 1980s, nalidixic acid was officially listed as a cancer-causing drug. [1] Variations on the nalidixic acid molecule created new compounds called the quinolones, which in turn were given catchy names by the pharmaceutical companies—thus we know quinolones as the "floxin" drugs. [2]

Quinolones work by inhibiting the bacterial chemical responsible for unwinding and copying DNA. They are used to treat upper respiratory infections, bronchitis, hospital-acquired pneumonia, urinary tract infections, complicated intra-abdominal infection, prostate infections, and infections of the skin, bones, and joints. In addition, there are three special uses of quinolones: to treat exposure to inhaled anthrax powder (as an alternative to tetracycline), treating the plague, and treatment of cancer patients who have fever with low white cell counts. Because they interfere with DNA copying, quinolones are being investigated for use as anticancer agents. [3]

The quinolones came into more frequent use with the rise of antibiotic resistance to other drugs. There are now four later generations of quinolones, and they differ from nalidixic acid in several respects, especially the presence of a fluorine atom on the later drugs. "Flox-" (for fluorine) is a part of all of their chemical names. Several of the later generation drugs also have significant toxicities.

There are six main quinolones in use today:

> ciprofloxacin (Cipro, Cipro XR, Ciprobay, Ciproxin, Ciloxan Ophthalmic)
>
> levofloxacin (Levaquin, Cravit, Quixin Ophthalmic)
>
> moxifloxacin (Avelox, Vigamox)
>
> ofloxacin (Floxin, Ocuflox, Floxin Otic, Optiflox, Oxaldin, Tarivid)
>
> norfloxacin (Norxin)
>
> gemifloxacin (Factive)

The US drug approval system requires drug makers to submit safety and effectiveness information in four phases:

1. phase 1 tests the drug on a limited number of healthy people;

2. phase 2 tests the drug on a small number of people with infections that the antibiotic is actively treating;

3. phase 3 tests the drug on larger numbers of ill persons.

After phase 3, the drug is approved and marketed.

4. Phase 4 is not testing—it is mandatory reporting by the company to the FDA of all the information it collected from patients and doctors about adverse drug effects.

Temafloxacin went through phases 1, 2, and 3 and was approved, then removed from the market after only three months due to 50 reports of severe adverse reactions, including three deaths. It caused dangerously low blood sugar, kidney failure, destruction of red blood cells, liver injury, and life threatening hypersensitivity reactions. Grepafloxacin was introduced to the market in 1997 and withdrawn in 1999 due to reports of severe cardiovascular events. While all quinolones can cause heart problems, the frequency and severity caused by grepafloxacin could not be predicted based on the relatively small number of test subjects required by the FDA for approval.

Lomefloxacin was approved before it was evident just how severely phototoxic it could be—that was not appreciated until it was in broad use. Some patients on lomefloxacin can get blistering skin reactions from slight ultraviolet light exposure, even when it is just light that comes through glass windows while indoors, or outdoors in shade. The drug is still available as a generic, but rarely used.

Trovafloxacin was another approved quinolone, this one causing severe liver damage and dangerously low blood sugar. In the United States and Canada, the drug can only be used in the hospital for treatment of serious life – or limb-threatening infections. [4]

As these four drug stories illustrate, one should never be the first to try a drug that is relatively new to the market. It is wise to wait at least two years to allow time for the true severity and magnitude of adverse drug effects to become evident in "phase 4" reports to the FDA. While the extreme toxicity of these four quinolones have been especially recognized, any of the other drugs in this class have the potential for similar adverse effects.

Many bacteria have figured out how to resist the effect of quinolones by changing the structure of the enzyme targeted by the drugs, or stiffening up the defenses in their outer walls to make it harder for the drug to penetrate the cell, and by developing a pump that funnels the drug out of the cell. The use of quinolones was so widespread in poultry farming that a common bacteria causing diarrhea in chickens and humans became totally resistant to the drugs. This prompted the US government to mandate the end of routine quinolone use in poultry manufacture in order to preserve drug effectiveness in humans. [5]

Quinolones are eliminated mostly through the kidneys, so they have to be used with extreme caution in people who already have kidney trouble.

Urine should be kept acidic, and plenty of fluids are needed so as to avoid crystals forming in the urine.

The most frequent adverse reactions of quinolones are nausea, diarrhea, abnormal liver function tests, vomiting, and rash. Quinolone treatment could result in the usual antibiotic side effect of C difficile associated profuse, watery diarrhea and severe colon inflammation. Quinolones tend to block the junction of nerve and muscle. They can worsen the disease myasthenia gravis by paralyzing breathing muscles and causing death. People who are hypersensitive to quinolones could get fever, rash, or severe life-threatening skin reactions with blistering and peeling. Other hypersensitivity reactions include inflammation of the blood vessels, joint and muscle pain, lung inflammation, kidney failure, liver failure, and severe anemia.

Since the structure of quinolones is unlike any other class of antibiotic, they have some unique adverse effects. The package inserts carry Black Box warnings for tendon rupture. Quinolones can cause inflammation and possible tearing of tendons at any place in the body where connective tissue attaches muscle to bone. The Achilles tendon at the back of the heel is most frequently involved, and if it tears straight through, an operation is needed for repair. Other frequent sites of tendon injury are the shoulder (rotator cuff), hand, biceps, thumb, and wrist. Tendon damage from quinolones is common in children and people over 60, those on steroids, organ transplant patients, and people with rheumatoid arthritis. It can happen within the first two days on the drug or be delayed until months after quinolone treatment. Quinolones can cause juvenile rheumatoid arthritis in children with severe pain and weakness. In children, the drugs are only approved for treatment of the plague or for exposure to inhaled anthrax powder.

Although all antibiotics have the possibility of causing some mental effects, they can be particularly severe with quinolones. Stephen Fried wrote *Bitter Pills: Inside the Hazardous World of Legal Drugs* to tell the story of his wife's severe mental distortion after taking just one Floxin pill. The doctor told her it was a new wonder drug and prescribed it to treat a urinary tract infection so minor she didn't even know she had it.

Six hours after taking one pill, she was delirious. The quinolone drugs can cause so-called toxic psychosis, meaning insanity caused by a poison. In addition to acting on the brain, quinolones can cause malfunction of the nerves going to the body. The nerve damage can be permanent. [6]

Quinolone effects on the brain, nerves, and mental functions can include:

restlessness	irrational fears
dizziness	feeling not oneself (depersonalization)
lightheadedness	depression
insomnia	suicide
nightmares	numbness and tingling
hallucinations	burning pain
manic reaction	sharp, jabbing pain
paranoia	electric-like pain
irritability	extreme touch sensitivity
tremor	lack of coordination
inability to walk	heat intolerance
muscle weakness	paralysis
weakness	drowsiness

convulsive seizures (including a seizure that won't stop on its own)

Despite the change in warnings on the package insert since 2004, there continues to be a high incidence of peripheral neuropathy reported to the FDA Adverse Event Reporting System. The true incidence of mental effects is unknown since many physicians are not aware of these possible effects or are reluctant to admit their prescription could have caused such devastating problems. Patients are not likely to realize and report a possible drug connection to their doctors, and instead end up in the hands of a psychiatrist.

Other potential adverse effects of quinolones:

abdominal pain	shortness of breath
foot pain	swelling of breathing passages
pain in extremities	fluid on lungs
skin, hair, or nail changes	bloody nose

palpitation

irregular heart beat

delayed electrical conduction in heart

blacking out

high or low blood pressure

chest pain (angina pectoris)

heart attack (myocardial infarction)

sudden death (cardiopulmonary arrest)

blood clot in brain (stroke)

painful in mouth from overgrowth of yeast

painful swallowing

ruptured intestines

internal bleeding

yellow jaundice

liver inflammation and liver failure

inflammation of pancreas

swollen lymph nodes

bleeding under skin

joint pain and stiffness

back pain

gout flare up

muscle weakness

kidney inflammation and injury

kidney failure

inability to urinate

frequent urination

blood in urine

crystals in urine

inflamed vagina

breast pain

breast enlargement

hiccough

wheezing

blood clot in lungs

itching

welt-like hives

severe sensitivity to sun and UV rays

flushing

fever

chills

swelling of face, neck, and tongue

overgrowth of yeast on skin

darkening of skin

sweating

blurred vision

change in color perception

over brightness of lights

blurry vision

double vision

eye pain

erratic jerking of eyes

ringing in ears

hearing loss

bad taste in mouth

anemia

low white blood cells

low platelets

high blood sugar

low blood sugar

depletions of vitamins B2, B9, B12

depletion of biotin

depletion of vitamin K

depletion of zinc [7, 8, 9]

Quinolones are assigned pregnancy category C since there are insufficient studies to demonstrate their safe use while pregnant.

Quinolones are partially processed through the liver and can aggravate the side effects of any other drug sharing the same metabolic pathway. They can delay the electrical conduction in the heart and are more likely to cause damage when given at the same time as other drugs that delay heart conduction. Quinolones should not be given with drugs that interfere with the neuro-muscular junction, making paralysis more likely.

Possible drug interactions include:

theophylline	clozapine (Clozaril)
tizanidine (Zanaflex)	anti-inflammatory drugs (Advil, Motrin)
oral diabetic drugs	sildenafil (Viagra)
phenytoin (Dilantin)	caffeine
cyclosporine	duloxetine (Cymbalta)
blood thinners	probenecid
methotrexate	lidocaine [7, 8, 9]
ropinirole (Requip)	

Overuse of the quinolones has led to such widespread bacterial resistance that they are now only appropriate for mild to moderate infections in persons who are not in danger of dying from a simple infection. On the other hand, why risk any of these awful side effects for a non-life-threatening condition in the first place?

CHAPTER 14

MISCELLANEOUS ANTIBIOTICS

Metronidazole (Flagyl)

Metronidazole is a synthetic chemical in a class of its own. It works by damaging the DNA of bacteria and parasites. It causes cancerous tumors to grow in laboratory animals. In humans, it increases the risk of cancer in Crohn's disease patients. It is known to cross the placental barrier and pass into breast milk, therefore it is not allowed in the first trimester of pregnancy or in breastfeeding women. It easily penetrates into the brain and all tissues, so its side effects can be severe:

stumbling

dizziness

difficulty speaking

seizures

poisoning the nerves

vision problems

numbness

tingling

seizures

blackouts

meningitis

headache

incoordination

furry tongue

tongue inflammation

mouth inflammation

sudden overgrowth of *Candida*

rash

itching

hives

skin peeling

dead skin

nose congestion

dry mouth

dry vagina

fever

confusion	low white cell count
depression	low platelet count
weakness	changes on EKG tracing
insomnia	painful urination
disorientation	inflamed bladder
nausea	loss of bladder control
lack of appetite	darkened urine
vomiting	vaginal yeast infection
diarrhea	joint pains
stomach pain	loss of sexual desire
cramping	painful intercourse
constipation	fungal superinfections [1]
metallic taste	

Metronidazole interacts with many drugs and should not be taken with lithium, blood thinners, busulfan, or any drug inhibiting metronidazole breakdown in the liver. If someone drinks alcohol while on this drug, they will get belly cramps, nausea, vomiting, headaches, and flushing. In alcoholic patients taking disulfiram, concurrent use of metronidazole can cause a psychotic reaction.

Alternatives to Flagyl for treating vaginal trichomonas infections include garlic suppositories, echinacea, goldenseal, barberry, myrrh, and tea tree oil. [2]

Nitrofurans

Nitrofurans include only two common drugs:

1. Nitrofurantoin (Macrodantin, Macrobid, Furadantin) for urinary tract infection

2. Furazolidone (Furoxone, Dependal-M. Diafuron, medaron) for diarrhea caused by bacteria or parasites.

Nitrofurantoin is an entirely man made molecule, first approved for use in the United States in 1953. The drug concentrates in the bladder, where it can be very effective against bacteria causing urinary tract infections (UTIs). The basic chemical structure of the nitrofurans is related to the anti-seizure drug phenytoin, the muscle relaxant drug dantrolene, and the insecticide imiprothrin. [3]

Nitrofuran seems to work against bacteria, parasites, and insects by undergoing reactions that produce free radicals—these are unstable and highly reactive molecules that are extremely damaging to DNA, to the protein-making machinery of cells, and to cell walls. Free radicals cause molecular 'holes' in an action similar to rust eroding metal. This works great to kill bacteria, but it also could cause considerable collateral damage to the body's cells.

The common side effects of nitrofurans are:

nausea	dizziness
diarrhea	drowsiness
indigestion	rash

The drugs can also cause:

loss of appetite	vomiting
joint pains	gas
chest pains	weakness
fever and chills	headache
shortness of breath	bluish lips and fingers
cough	itching
stomach upset	discolored urine

Macrobid and related drugs can cause rare side effects that patients should be aware of because they are very severe. These include a scarring condition of the lungs called pulmonary fibrosis, for which there is no very effective treatment short of lung transplant. Nitrofurans can cause peripheral neuropathy, where the nerves are painful or there is numbness. They can cause severe skin inflammation resulting in massive skin shedding that looks similar to burns. Nitrofurans can cause the body to attack its own red blood cells, resulting in anemia that is untreatable even with transfusions. These drugs can cause vasculitis, where the body attacks its own blood vessels; lupus, with skin changes; joint pain; and kidney damage. Nitrofurans are one of the most common causes of drug-induced liver damage and should not be given to anyone with a history of yellow jaundice. The liver damage can be severe and lead to liver failure or cirrhosis.

These serious adverse effects are more likely to happen in people who are on long-term nitrofurans, such as for suppression of recurrent urinary tract infections. They all have in common the phenomenon of auto-immunity, meaning the drugs somehow provoke the body into attacking its own tissue.

The DNA-damaging effects of nitrofurans make these drugs capable of causing cancer (carcinogenic). Animal studies have shown an excess of breast cancer and ovarian cancer in animals exposed to nitrofurans. These drugs are used in livestock animals in many non-US countries. The residues of nitrofurans do not degrade to a significant extent upon cooking, baking, grilling, and microwaving, so the carcinogenic drug residues persist in food eaten by humans. According to the US Government Office of Technology Assessment, "Thus there is probably no level at which it is absolutely safe." [4]

Despite what is known about the cancer causing potential, nitrofurans that are used as pesticides have no assignment of so-called "maximum residue levels" considered safe to humans. Scientists have not determined what the maximum acceptable daily intake might be. [5]

The US bans use of nitrofurans in homegrown livestock and imported seafood. As recently as November 2015, the government was seizing and destroying shipments of nitrofuran-treated seafood imports that originated in India, Indonesia, and Malaysia. [6]

As with all antibiotics, the nitrofurans can destroy the normal balance of beneficial bacteria in the gut, leading to overgrowth of Clostridium difficile bacteria and resultant bloody diarrhea. Nitrofuran antibiotics can lead to infection with super-resistant bacteria that have developed mechanisms to avoid the medication's effects. Nitrofurans cross the placenta and enter breast milk. They are not to be used close to delivery or while breastfeeding. Nitrofurans interact with many other drugs, so all medications should be discussed in full with the doctor and pharmacist before taking this drug. [7]

Macrobid was popular for the treatment of urinary tract infections, but its toxicities made the drug only third or fourth choice once amoxicillin came on the market in 1970, followed rapidly by the introduction of several other new antibiotics. The cephalosporins (like Keflex) and quinolone drugs (like Cipro) have become other likely options to treat UTIs. But the emergence of antibiotic resistance against the newer drugs is causing Macrobid to make a strong comeback. Serious adverse events will become more prevalent when this class of drugs begins to get overused again.

Rifaximin (Xifaxan)

Rifaximin is used to treat the most common cause of traveler's diarrhea, a certain strain of E coli bacteria that produces a toxin. Enterotoxigenic E coli, or ETEC, produces a toxin that can cause massive diarrhea and rarely leads to kidney failure. There are four other common bacterial causes of traveler's diarrhea that rifaximin does not help with. If rifaximin is taken without having had a stool sample tested, then it is likely that the drug itself will only cause more diarrhea—while treating nothing. The fact is that most cases of traveler's diarrhea, regardless of the kind of infecting bacteria, will resolve without drug treatment in 3 to 5 days. Rifaximin is for longer lasting cases or for when the patient is severely ill with extreme dehydration, severe electrolyte derangements, and high fever. Rifaximin is also used to treat irritable bowel symptoms, which can be distressing but are often not worth the risk of adverse drug effects. Rifaximin is sometimes given to patients with cirrhosis to kill off the ammonia-producing in the colon; this decreases buildup of ammonia and reduced the tendency of cirrhotic patients to develop mental symptoms.

Common adverse reactions to rifaximin are:

swelling   belly pain
nausea   anemia

dizziness	depression
fatigue	joint pain
fluid buildup in abdomen	shortness of breath
muscle spasms	fever

Like other antibiotics, rifaximin can cause overgrowth of C difficile resulting in colitis and bloody diarrhea. It can promote the development of super-resistant bacteria. [8]

Vancomycin

Vancomycin is a naturally occurring antibiotic produced by bacteria originally collected in the tropical jungle of Borneo (an island in the South China Sea). Its name derives from the word vanquish, implying effectiveness in eradicating infections. Vancomycin is given intravenously to treat serious infections caused by a strain of *Staphylococcus aureus* that is resistant to methicillin, called MRSA. This includes MRSA infections of bone, heart valves, blood stream, and brain (meningitis). Each dose of vancomycin IV must be infused very slowly over no less than a full hour in order to avoid Red Man Syndrome, where the patient flushes red and gets swelling of the lips and throat possibly leading to shock.

When a patient on another antibiotic gets colitis and bloody diarrhea from overgrowth of C difficile, often it is enough to simply stop the drug. If colitis continues, it is necessary to treat with vancomycin given orally as Vancocin so that it can work directly on the bowel. Vancomycin can cause kidney and ear toxicity, and this is more likely to occur when the patient already has some kidney disease or other drugs toxic to the kidneys are given concurrently. Vancomycin causes low white blood cell count and low platelets.

Serious side effects of vancomycin include kidney failure and hearing loss. Vancomycin is very irritating to tissues and should be slowly infused when it is given by vein. Vancomycin is given by mouth to treat antibiotic-associated C difficile diarrhea, but if the colon is highly inflamed, then the vancomycin could be absorbed and reach toxic blood levels. Other potential adverse effects include low white blood cell count, vein inflammation, allergic reaction, drug fever, and blistering skin eruption. [9]

Linezolid (Zyvox)

When vancomycin causes colitis or when it fails to effectively treat colitis or MRSA, the drug of choice is linezolid (Zyvox). Zyvox blocks the first step in bacterial protein manufacture. But, Zyvox can cause low platelets, making bleeding possible. It can cause nerve pain or numbness and interferes with how the body handles serotonin. Zyvox can cause serotonin syndrome, a particular set of bizarre psychiatric disturbances with drastic physical signs that can be life-threatening: agitation, hallucinations, unstable heart rate, unstable blood pressure, very high temperature, abnormal neurologic reflexes, incoordination, nausea, vomiting, and diarrhea. In severe cases, it can progress to coma and death. Serotonin syndrome can occur when taking a single drug, but is especially likely when more than one drug affecting serotonin is used at the same time. For this reason, Zyvox should not be given to patients on antidepressants. [10]

Pfizer was in hot water with the FDA when they were found to be aggressively promoting Zyvox to doctors for use in all kinds of infections well beyond what it was FDA-approved for. The company continued to advertise it for other conditions even after an FDA warning letter, selling $4.4 billion worth of Zyvox in an eight-year period. Finally, the US Department of Justice (DOJ) joined a whistleblower lawsuit to bring fraud charges against the company. The charges included promoting Zyvox for the treatment of catheter related skin and bloodstream infections. In fact, the Zyvox package insert describes a significantly increased death rate in patients with this type of infection.

Other charges in the lawsuit were for making false claims promoting Zyvox for the treatment of surgical site infections, prevention of surgical site infections, treating MRSA when vancomycin could be used, and claiming to be superior to vancomycin. The drug was only FDA-approved for use when an infection was resistant to vancomycin. Pfizer went so far as to promote Zyvox as the drug of choice for any infection, anywhere, even though it has only been proven to work against certain bacteria. Additionally, the DOJ found that Pfizer even paid health care professionals to promote its off-label uses, in violation of federal anti-kickback laws.

This false advertising was not simply a profit maker for Pfizer, but put the entire world at risk of losing an important antibiotic. As of today, Zyvox is the drug to use when vancomycin fails to work. If Zyvox were to be used loosely, in the way Pfizer illegally promoted it, then antibiotic resistance would surely develop very quickly. The FDA had this concern in mind when it specifically approved Zyvox for only those infections caused by vancomycin-resistant bacteria. In 2009, Pfizer agreed to pay $2.3 billion to settle the DOJ charges, and that included $1 billion for illegal marketing of four drugs, including Zyvox. [11] That $2.3 billion settlement was the largest healthcare fraud settlement to date.

Lincosamides

The Lincosamide drugs were named after Lincoln, Nebraska where the soil organism that secretes this antibiotic came from. These drugs prevent bacteria from replicating by interfering with how they make proteins. The original drug, lincocin, was chemically manipulated to create clindamycin, a more powerful antibiotic used as an eye ointment for conjunctivitis.

Clindamycin (Cleocin) is one of the most likely of the antibiotics to cause colitis, along with the cephalosporins, fluoroquinolones, and extended-coverage penicillins. One study of patients on clindamycin showed the incidence of stomach upset was about 21%, diarrhea occurred in 13%, and colitis in 2.3%. [12] Clindamycin rarely causes a life threatening skin reaction. In children it has caused "gasping syndrome" due to the benzoyl alcohol preservative. Clindamycin should be reserved for the most seriously ill hospitalized patients with Staph pneumonia, for Strep infections in penicillin allergic patients, and for infections by organisms that thrive in a low oxygen environment, such as the bug responsible for gangrene. [13] Clindamycin also comes in a topical preparation for acne. A small amount is absorbed through the skin, so the topical form only causes colitis in less than 1% of users. Clindamycin also treats some parasitic infections, including malaria.

Drugs to Treat Tuberculosis (TB)

There are at least a dozen drugs to treat TB, and typically, two or more drugs are prescribed at once because drug resistance is such a pervasive problem. If a person only takes one TB drug, the species of bacteria they are infected with will rapidly mutate and become resistant. Treatment for patients with first-time TB consists of a 2-month regimen of isoniazid (INH), rifampicin, pyrazinamide, and ethambutol simultaneously, followed by 4 months of INH with rifampicin. [14]

INH disrupts the construction of the bacterial cell wall. It can cause rashes, liver irritation progressing to severe liver injury and cirrhosis, and severe stomach discomfort with nausea and vomiting.

Ethambutol disrupts the construction of the bacterial cell wall and is uniquely toxic to the eye nerves, resulting in optic neuritis with loss of vision. It can also cause rashes.

Pyrazinamide works by disrupting the membrane separating the cell wall from the bacterium's innards and blocks the cell's energy production. It can cause rashes, liver irritation progressing to severe liver injury and cirrhosis, stomach upset, joint pain, rash, gout, and kidney stones.

Rifampin interferes with the mechanisms the bacteria uses to manufacture proteins. It can cause rashes; liver irritation progressing to severe liver injury and cirrhosis; flu like symptoms half a day after the dose with fever, fatigue, headache, and body aches; low platelet count, which makes it hard to clot blood normally; and/or an allergic reaction resulting in damage to the kidneys; reddish-orange tint to the sweat, tears, and urine.

Isoniazid can cause nerve damage with numbness and burning of toes and fingers and interacts with the amino acid tyramine naturally occurring in foods such as red wine and aged cheese, causing flushing and palpitations. It can cause confusion psychosis, insomnia, headache, lupus-like symptoms of joint pains and fever, fatigue, and weight loss.

Patients with drug resistant TB are treated with drug combinations consisting of three to five drugs. These can include the first-line drugs listed above, plus any combination of the following:

- IV medications such as the aminoglycosides (kanamycin, amikacin, capreomycin, and streptomycin)

- fluoroquinolones (levofloxacin, moxifloxacin, ofloxacin)

- para–aminosalicylic acid

- cycloserine, or its derivative terizidone

- thionamide drugs (ethionamide prothionamide)

Para-aminosalicylic acid (brand name Paser) works against TB by inhibiting the way bacteria make the B vitamin folate and inhibiting the bacteria from taking up iron. The most common side effects are nausea, vomiting, diarrhea, and abdominal pain. Paser can cause liver damage, signaled by rash, fever, and/or jaundice, which can be deadly. It can cause chromosome damage and abnormalities in the unborn baby. It can cause autoimmune reactions, where the body attacks itself, resulting in fevers, swollen lymph nodes, low white cell count making the patient susceptible to infections, low platelet count and clotting ability, anemia, inflammation of the heart lining and blood vessels, low blood sugar, damage to eye nerves, and brain inflammation. [15]

Cycloserine and its derivative terizidone can cause heart failure and rashes, but their most severe toxic effects are on the nervous system. They can cause convulsions, drowsiness, headache, tremor, difficulty speaking, dizziness, confusion with disorientation and loss of memory, psychosis with suicidal tendencies, irritability, aggression, severe depression, anxiety, panic attacks, paranoia, seeing and hearing things that don't exist, weakness of arms and legs, numbness, and coma. [16]

The thioamide drugs (ethionamide and prothionamide) cause stomach upset and can be toxic to the liver. They can cause acne, allergic reactions, hair loss, convulsions, dermatitis, double vision, dizziness, headache, low blood pressure, numbness and pain in nerves, and joint pains. [17]

Topical Antibiotics

The most common brands of topical antibiotics are Bacitracin, Neosporin, Polymyxin B, and Triple Antibiotic Ointment. Topical antibiotics are generally very well tolerated. The most common side effects are skin irritation or minor rash, but hives and severe allergic reactions are possible. Serious adverse effects are rare but can include:

abnormal heart rhythm	seizures
low blood pressure	slow heartbeat
drowsiness	toxic effect on brain or spinal cord
head pains	toxicity to organs of hearing
involuntary quivering	turning blue
lung failure causing loss of breath	unconsciousness

There are several effective alternatives to commercial topical antibiotics. Silver has been used as a topical wound-healing mineral for over 3000 years. It is spectacularly effective for minor skin infections as well as major conditions such as diabetic wounds and burns. [18] Raw honey can be a very effective treatment for open wounds, with Manuka honey (from the New Zealand Manuka flower) being the most studied for specific antibacterial action. [19] You can make an herbal ointment using coconut oil as a base, or make a liquid that uses almond oil, grapeseed oil, or olive oil as a base. Add anti-bacterial herbs such as chamomile, plantain, lavender, calendula, tea tree oil, or comfrey, to name just a few common western herbs. Thicken the mixture by adding beeswax. [20]

CHAPTER 15

Consumer Beware

The average health care consumer can protect against "over prescribing" and unnecessary adverse drug effects for them self and their loved ones.

First and foremost, abandon the notion that every sign of illness needs to be answered with a prescription. It is a simple matter of not putting yourself in harm's way unnecessarily by popping a pill that doesn't benefit you. Equally important is to look at your lifestyle habits and environment to prevent poor health situations by avoiding products that place convenience and seller profit margins over concern for health or safety risks.

Secondly, remember that your doctor works for you. You may have no choice but to pay for government-mandated insurance and fork over the deductible and co-pays, but don't relinquish responsibility for decisions around accepting questionable diagnoses in the absence of simple testing and don't blindly accept antibiotic prescriptions just because they "might" help. The prevailing healthcare model is strictly pharmaceutical and surgical. The typical five-to-seven minute doctor visit is entirely inadequate to thoroughly listen or provide counsel on non-drug alternatives. Cultivate the intention and habit of extracting what you need from the doctor's education and experience and actively participate in decision making about your own health. Above all, be alert that your expertise exceeds that of the doctor when it comes to your own health—no matter what a doctor might say or imply to the contrary.

Prescription drugs have effects other than the intended cure, particularly when there is more than one drug on board. Be aware of these effects so you can make informed decisions about your health care.

Remember the principles of Informed Consent. At the least, your doctor (or other prescribing health care provider) should be willing and able to answer these questions:

- Do you even have a bacterial infection?

- What is the recommended drug? What does it do?

- How well does the drug work for your specific condition?

- What is known about the antibiotic's side effects, including the 'Black Box Warnings' and other 'Special Precautions.'

- What are the alternatives to taking an antibiotic, including the expected result if you take no medicine at all?

- Is it being prescribed experimentally or off-label?

It is absolutely appropriate to demand a full physical and basic lab tests from your doctor, and it may also be prudent to seek an alternative practitioner for non-drug advice beyond the scope of training doctors practicing conventional medicine receive.

There are some additional, less obvious but more menacing situations that might be making you a victim of overprescribing habits. The usual doctor working in a practice with over 2,500 patients, seeing 30 patients a day, has little time or inclination to undertake a critical reading of his or her medical journals afterhours. So it is common practice to rely heavily on glossy promotional materials compiled by drug companies. Studies abundantly demonstrate that such advertising matter is misleading at best and criminally deceptive at worst. Yet pharmaceutical company advertising continues to be the primary, often *only*, medical "education" for too many physicians. This is heavily encouraged by the distribution of free sample medications, facilitating a real no-brainer for the clinic to give out a sample and follow up with a prescription. [1]

A diligent reading of select medical journals may not be much better, however. Most medical journals have some sort of conflict of interest policy that applies to authors, but the majority of such policies do not extend to disclosure of conflicts of interest for their reviewers, editors, or publishers. Even many of the non-profit physician organizations that publish journals often receive more revenue from advertising purchased in their journals than from membership fees. The fact is that journals would not be able to survive without advertising and medical journals whose editors too critically review studies sponsored by the drug industry can experience a substantial loss of advertising revenue. These problems led Richard Smith, editor with the *British Medical Journal* for 25 years, to conclude that medical journals are "an extension of the marketing arm of pharmaceutical companies." [2] It is wise never to underestimate the potential reach and influence of conflicts of interest, obvious or not.

Finally, it is completely reasonable for you to ask for full disclosure of your doctor's potential conflicts of interest. Typical conflicts of interest could include the clinic staff getting free lunches from the friendly drug sales reps, the doctor holding stock in pharmaceutical companies, or the medical center being paid to enroll patients in a drug study. Many medical offices are stocked with free samples, which encourages them to thoughtlessly give out the drug most readily at hand and follow it up with a very pricey prescription. If the doctor is writing with a pen emblazoned with a drug name, drinking from a coffee mug with a drug company logo, and writing on a pad with a drug logo, you know you are in a heavily influenced office.

Unfortunately, the Internet is even more saturated with advertising designed to support drug company interests first, consumer interests second or not at all. By actual survey, it's been reported that a product is being pushed directly or indirectly on 95% of consumer health sites. Sometimes it is evident by rolling your cursor over highlighted key words and watching ads pop up. Other times, you have to probe three clicks deep to see the pharma connection.

Above all, remember that you are the paying consumer, even though there is a Federal mandate to be insured (such as Obamacare). You have the right to expect doctors to work for you and that most definitely includes them answering your questions. If he or she does not have time or is offended, find another doctor pronto. In no circumstances should you give up your right to an opportunity for full informed consent. A smart consumer insists on being fully informed before agreeing to take any drug.

Thank you for your interest, and I hope you found the information helpful.

Please post your online review.

Please avail yourself of other books in the series:

No-Nonsense Guide to Psychiatric Drugs, Including Mental Effects of Common Non-Psych Medications

No-Nonsense Guide to Cholesterol Medications, Informed Consent and Statin Drugs

ABOUT THE AUTHOR

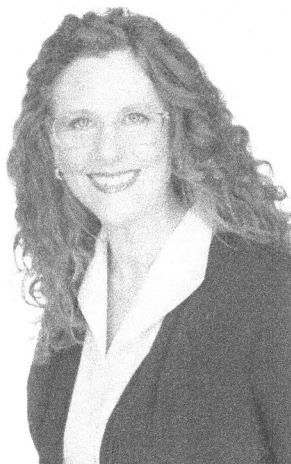

Moira Dolan, MD is a patient-centered physician and champion of Informed Consent, a graduate of the University of Illinois School of Medicine, and certified by the American Board of Internal Medicine as well as by the American Academy of Anti-Aging Medicine. For many years, Dr. Dolan consulted for the Office of the Inspector General in Texas to identify improper treatments and inappropriate medical billing claims, and she has served as Medical Director of a healthcare audit firm. She has no financial conflicts of interest for forwarding or censuring any particular drug treatment and intentionally sought out service providers for the packaging of this material who also did not have conflicts of interest. Dr. Dolan is director of The Medical Accountability Network and writes for the medical news blog on SmartMEDInfo.com. She lives in Austin, Texas.

ACKNOWLEDGEMENTS

I thank my esteemed colleague and good friend Eleanor McCulley, RN, of Austin 3D Health. She is the most knowledgeable and practical holistic practitioner I have ever worked with. Eleanor drove me to compose the No-Nonsense series in the first place, for the benefit of her patients, making sure to include answers to the most frequently asked questions she encounters. For this book, she shared with me the wisdom gained from years of experience in helping patients recover from a wide variety of antibiotic-induced deficits.

I am very fortunate to have as my editor Debra L Hartmann of IndieAuthorPublishingServices.com. Her suggestions are consistently in the direction of letting my passion for patient advocacy come through loud and clear. Her patient-oriented viewpoints constantly challenge me to be more direct and explain technical points in a way they can be easily understood. I am grateful to Debra for making me a better writer.

REFERENCES

Chapter 1

1. Shapiro, DJ, LA Hicks, AT Pavia, and AL Hersh. "Antibiotic prescribing for adults in ambulatory care in the USA, 2007-09". *J Antimicrob Chemother*. 2014 Jan;69(1):234-240.

2. Budnitz MD, MPH, Daniel S, Daniel A Pollock MD, Kelly N Weidenbach MPH, Aaron B Mendelsohn PhD MPH, Thomas J Schroeder MS, Joseph L Annest PhD. "National Surveillance of Emergency Department Visits for Outpatient Adverse Drug Events". *JAMA*. 2006;296(15):1858-1866.

3. Shehab, Nadine, Priti R Patel, Arjun Srinivasan, and Daniel S Budnitz. "Emergency department visits for antibiotic-associated adverse events". *Clin Infect Dis*. 2008;47(6):735-743.

4. Bourgeois, FT, KD Mandl, C Valim, and MW Shannon. "Pediatric adverse drug events in the outpatient setting: An 11-year national analysis". *Pediatrics*. 2009 Oct;124(4):e744-750.

5. World Health Organization. "Antimicrobial resistance, Fact sheet N°194". Updated April 2015 at http://www.who.int/mediacentre/factsheets/fs194/en/

6. Stephens, Pippa. "Antibiotic resistance now 'global threat', WHO warns". *BBC News*. 30 April 2014.

7. Shipley, David. "Fight to Save Antibiotics". *Bloomberg View*

Editorial. June 2, 2016. https://www.bloomberg.com/view/articles/2016-06-02/fight-to-save-antibiotics

8. Rodgers, Paul. "Antibiotic 'Apocalypse' Feared". *Forbes.com*. May 23, 2014. http://www.forbes.com/sites/paulrodgers/2014/05/23/fears-for-antibiotic-apocalypse-grow/#246bbbdb5ad9

9. Kristensen, Malene Lopez, Palle Mark Christensen, and Jesper Hallas. "The effect of statins on average survival in randomised trials, an analysis of end point postponement". *BMJ Open*. 2015 Sep 24;5(9)e007118.

10. Jones, W H S, translator of Hippocrates' *Ancient Medicine. Airs, Waters, Places. Epidemics 1 and 3. The Oath. Precepts. Nutriment.* Loeb Classical Libraries, 1923.

Chapter 2

1. Jeters, RT, GR Wang, K Moon, NB Shoemaker, AA Salyers. "Tetracycline-associated transcriptional regulation of transfer genes of the Bacteroides conjugative transposon CTnDOT". *J Bacteriol*. 2009 Oct;191(20): 6374–6382.

2. Schaechter, Moselio, Robert Kolter, and Merry Buckley. "Microbiology in the 21st Century: Where Are We and Where Are We Going?". *American Academy of Microbiology*. 2004. Available at: http://academy.asm.org/index.php/general-microbiology/450-microbiology-in-the-21st-century-where-are-we-and-where-are-we-going.

3. Harrison, Laird. "Antibiotics Still Overprescribed for Sore Throats, Bronchitis". *Medscape*. Oct 04, 2013.

4. "Antibiotic Resistance Threats in the United States, 2013". *CDC*. Apr 2013. http://www.cdc.gov/drugresistance/threat-report-2013/index.html.

5. McGann, Patrick, Erik Snesrud, Rosslyn Maybank, et al. "*Escherichia coli* Harboring *mcr-1* and *bla*CTX-M on a Novel

IncF Plasmid: First report of *mcr-1* in the USA". Antimicrobial Agents and Chemotherapy, 2016.

6. Zhang, Sarah. "A Woman Was Killed by a Superbug Resistant to All 26 American Antibiotics, She won't be the last". The Atlantic, Jan 13, 2017.

7. "Office-Related Antibiotic Prescribing for Persons Aged ≤14 Years — United States, 1993-1994 to 2007-2008". *CDC*. Morb Mortal Wkly Rep: Sep 3, 2011;60(34);1153-1156.

8. US Food and Drug Administration Press Release: "FDA issues proposed rule to determine safety and effectiveness of antibacterial soaps". *FDA*. December 16, 2013.

9. Natural Resources Defense Council Press Release: "Triclosan Exposure Levels Increasing in Humans, New Data Shows Potential for Food Contamination". *NRDC*. August 5, 2010.

10. Nongmaithem, Jiten Singh, Dongkyu Shin, Han Myoung Lee, Hyun Tae Kim, Ho-Jin Chang, Joong Myung Cho, Kwang S Kim, Seonggu Ro. "Structural basis of triclosan resistance". *Journal of Structural Biology*. Nov 2010;174(1):173-179.

11. Tavernise, Sabrina. "Antibiotics in Livestock: F.D.A. Finds Use Is Rising". *NY Times*. Oct. 2, 2014.

12. Berkelman, RL. "Human illness associated with use of veterinary vaccines". *Clin Infect Dis*. 2003 Aug 1;37(3):407-414.

13. Kupferschmidt, Kai. "Chicken Vaccines Combine to Produce Deadly Virus". *ScienceNow*. 12 July 2012. http://www.sciencemag.org/news/2012/07/chicken-vaccines-combine-produce-deadly-virus.

14. Sarmah, AK, MT Meyer, and AB Boxall. "A global perspective on the use, sales, exposure pathways, occurrence, fate and effects of veterinary antibiotics (VAs) in the environment". *Chemosphere*. 2006 Oct;65(5):725–759.

15. Devries, Mark. Video of stealth drone over a pig farm: http://factoryfarmdrones.com/.

16. Done, HY and RU Halden. "Reconnaissance of 47 antibiotics and associated microbial risks in seafood sold in the United States". *J Hazard Mater*. 2015 Jan 23;282:10-17

17. Done, HY, AK Venkatesan, and RU Halden. "Does the Recent Growth of Aquaculture Create Antibiotic Resistance Threats Different from those Associated with Land Animal Production in Agriculture?". *AAPS J*. 2015 May;17(3):513-524.

18. Noah, Timothy. "The Make-Believe Billion: How drug companies exaggerate research costs to justify absurd profits". *Slate.com*. Mar 3, 2011. http://www.slate.com/articles/business/the_customer/2011/03/the_makebelieve_billion.html

19. Anderson, Richard. "Pharmaceutical industry gets high on fat profits". *BBC News*. 6 November 2014. http://www.bbc.com/news/business-28212223

20. Aydin, S, B Ince, and O Ince. "Development of antibiotic resistance genes in microbial communities during long-term operation of anaerobic reactors in the treatment of pharmaceutical wastewater". *Water Res*. 2015 Oct 15;83:337-344.

21. Xi, Chuanwu, Yongli Zhang, Carl F Marrs, Wen Ye, Carl Simon, Betsy Foxman, Jerome Nriagu. "Prevalence of Antibiotic Resistance in Drinking Water Treatment and Distribution Systems". *Appl Environ Microbiol*. September 2009; 75(17):5714-5718.

22. Vaz-Moreira, Ivone, Olga C Nunes, Célia M Manaia. "Bacterial diversity and antibiotic resistance in water habitats: searching the links with the human microbiome". *FEMS Microbiology Reviews*. Jul 2014;38(4):761–778.

23. Yi, T, TG Kim, and KS Cho. "Fate and behavior of extended-spectrum β-lactamase-producing genes in municipal sewage

treatment plants". *J Environ Sci Health A Tox Hazard Subst Environ Eng.* 2015;50(11):1160-1168.

24. Bollinger, RR, AS Barbas, EL Bush, SS Lin, and W Parker. "Biofilms in the normal human large bowel: fact rather than fiction". *Gut.* 2007 Oct;56(10)"1481-1482.

25. *Nutrition and Oral Medicine*, edited by Riva Touger-Decker, Connie Mobley, Joel B Epstein. Humana Press (2014).

26. Niazi, SA, D Clark, T Do, SC Gilbert, F Foschi, F Mannocci, D Beighton. "The effectiveness of enzymic irrigation in removing a nutrient-stressed endodontic multispecies biofilm". *Int Endod J.* 2014 Aug;47(8):756-768.

27. Watters, CM, T Burton, DK Kirui, NJ Millenbaugh. "Enzymatic degradation of in vitro Staphylococcus aureus biofilms supplemented with human plasma". *Infect Drug Resist.* 2016 Apr 27;9:71-78.

28. Sakoulas, G, GP Wormser, P Visintainer, WS Aronow, RB Nadelman. "Relationship between population density of attorneys and prevalence of methicillin-resistant Staphylococcus aureus: is medical-legal pressure on physicians a driving force behind the development of antibiotic resistance?". *Am J Ther.* 2009 Sep-Oct;16(5):e1-6.

Chapter 3

1. Dubos, René Jules. *Man, Medicine, and Environment.* New York; Washington; London: F A Praeger, 1968.

2. Yano, Jessica M, Kristie Yu, Gregory P Donaldson, Gauri G Shastri, Phoebe Ann, et al. "Indigenous Bacteria from the Gut Microbiota Regulate Host Serotonin Biosynthesis". *Cell.* 9 Apr 2015;161(2):264–276.

3. Nezami, Behtash Ghazi and Shanthi Srinivasan. "Enteric Nervous System in the Small Intestine: Pathophysiology

and Clinical Implications". *Curr Gastroenterol Rep*. 2010 Oct;12(5):358–365.

4. De Palma, G, SM Collins, P Bercik, and EF Verdu. "The microbiota–gut–brain axis in gastrointestinal disorders: stressed bugs, stressed brain or both?". *J Physiol*. 2014 Jul 15;592(14):2989–2997.

5. Banerjee, S and JT Lamont. "Non-antibiotic therapy for Clostridium difficile infection". *Curr Opin Infect Dis*. 2000 Jun;13(3):215-219.

6. Kelesidis, T and C Pothoulakis. "Efficacy and safety of the probiotic Saccharomyces boulardii for the prevention and therapy of gastrointestinal disorders". *Therap Adv Gastroenterol*. 2012 Mar;5(2):111–125.

Chapter 4

1. Bisno, AL. "Are Cephalosporins Superior to Penicillin for Treatment of Acute Streptococcal Pharyngitis?". *Clin Infect Dis*. 2004 Jun 1;38(11):1535-1537.

2. Pichichero, ME, SM Marsocci, ML Murphy, W Hoeger, JL Green, A Sorrento. "Incidence of streptococcal carriers in private pediatric practice". *Arch Pediatr Adolesc Med*. 1999 Jun;153(6):624-628.

3. Tepes, B, A O'Connor, JP Gisbert, and C O'Morain. "Treatment of Helicobacter pylori infection 2012". *Helicobacter*. 2012 Sep;17 Suppl 1:36-42.

4. Rahnama, M, D Mehrabani, S Japoni, M Edjtehadi, and M Saberi Firoozi. "The healing effect of licorice (Glycyrrhiza glabra) on Helicobacter pylori infected peptic ulcers". *J Res Med Sci*. 2013 Jun;18(6):532–533.

5. Scott, D, D Weeks, K Melchers, and G Sachs. "The life and death of Helicobacter pylori". *Gut*. 1998 Jul;43 Suppl 1:S56–S60

6. Stover, Christy S and Christine M Litwin. "The Epidemiology of Upper Respiratory Infections at a Tertiary Care Center: Prevalence, Seasonality, and Clinical Symptoms". *Journal of Respiratory Medicine*. Vol. 2014, Article ID 469393, 8 pages.

7. CDC Flu Activity & Surveillance Page: http://www.cdc.gov/flu/weekly/fluactivitysurv.htm.

8. Chartrand, Caroline and Madhukar Pai. "How Accurate Are Rapid Influenza Diagnostic Tests?". Expert Rev Anti-Infect Ther. 2012;10(6):615-617.

9. "The Influenza Deception" by Brandon Turbeville. *The Activist Post*. January 21, 2014. http://www.activistpost.com/2014/01/the-influenza-deception.html.

10. Tamiflu label. Genentech, Inc, November 2014.

11. Williamson, IG, K Rumsby, S Benge, M Moore, PW Smith, M Cross, P Little. "Antibiotics and topical nasal steroid for treatment of acute maxillary sinusitis: a randomized controlled trial". *JAMA*. 2007 Dec 5;298(21):2487-2496.

12. Hickner, JM, JG Bartlett, RE Besser, R Gonzales, JR Hoffman, MA Sande. "Principles of Appropriate Antibiotic Use for Acute Rhinosinusitis in Adults: Background". *Ann of Intern Med*. 2001;134(6):498-505.

13. Lieberthal, Allan S, Aaron E Carroll, Tasnee Chonmaitree, Theodore G Ganiats, Alejandro Hoberman, Mary Anne Jackson, Mark D Joffe, Donald T Miller, Richard M Rosenfeld, Xavier D Sevilla, Richard H Schwartz, Pauline A Thomas, David E Tunkel. "The Diagnosis and Management of Acute Otitis Media". *Pediatrics*. March 1, 2013;131(3):e964 – e999.

14. "Summary Health Statistics Tables for US Adults: National Health Interview Survey, 2014" Table A-2. http://ftp.cdc.gov/pub/Health_Statistics/NCHS/NHIS/SHS/2014_SHS_Table_A-2.pdf AND "Pertussis Cases by Year" CDC Surveillance

and Reporting. http://www.cdc.gov/pertussis/surv-reporting/
cases-by-year.html#modalIdString_CDCTable_0

15. Mertsola MD, Jussi, He Qiushui MD. "*Bordetella pertussis*
(Whooping Cough) and other species". *AntiMicrobe.* http://
www.antimicrobe.org/b83-index.asp.

16. Dekker, AR, TJ Verheij, and AW van der Velden.
"Inappropriate antibiotic prescription for respiratory tract
indications: most prominent in adult patients". *Fam Pract.* 2015
Aug;32(4):401-407.

17. Sanchez, Guillermo V, Rebecca M Roberts, Alison P Albert,
Darcia D Johnson, Lauri A Hicks. "Effects of Knowledge,
Attitudes, and Practices of Primary Care Providers on Antibiotic
Selection, United States". *Emerging Infectious Diseases.* Dec
2014;20(12).

18. Linder MD, MPH, Jeffrey A, Jason N Doctor PhD, Mark
W Friedberg MD, MPP, Harry Reyes Nieva BA, Caroline Birks
MD, Daniella Meeker PhD, Craig R Fox PhD. "Time of Day
and the Decision to Prescribe Antibiotics". *JAMA Intern Med.*
2014;174(12):2029-2031.

19. Roumie, CL. "Inappropriate prescribing greatest in
nonphysician practitioners". *PharmacoEconomics & Outcomes
News.* August 2005;484(1):12-12.

20. Ahn, Ho-Young Anthony, Jin Seong Park, and Eric Haley.
"Consumers' Optimism Bias and Responses to Risk Disclosures
in Direct-to-Consumer (DTC) Prescription Drug Advertising:
The Moderating Role of Subjective Health Literacy". *Journal of
Consumer Affairs.* Mar 2014:48(1)175–194.

21. File Jr MD, Thomas M. "Antibiotic studies for the treatment
of community-acquired pneumonia in adults". *UpToDate.*
http://www.uptodate.com/contents/antibiotic-studies-for-
the-treatment-of-community-acquired-pneumonia-in-

adults?source=see_link&sectionName=DRUG+RESISTANCE
+AND+CHOICE+OF+THERAPY&anchor=H16#H16

22. McCutcheon, BA, DC Chang, LP Marcus, T Inui, A Noorbakhsh, C Schallhorn, R Parina, FR Salazar, MA Talamini. "Long-term outcomes of patients with non-surgically managed uncomplicated appendicitis". *J Am Coll Surg.* 2014 May;218(5):905–913.

23. Feingold, D, SR Steele, S Lee, A Kaiser, R Boushey, WD Buie, JF Rafferty. "Practice parameters for the treatment of sigmoid diverticulitis". *Dis Colon Rectum.* 2014 Mar;57(3):284-294.

24. Gordon, LB, MJ Waxman, L Ragsdale, and LS Mermel. "Overtreatment of presumed urinary tract infection in older women presenting to the emergency department". *J Am Geriatr Soc.* 2013 May;61(5):788-792.

25. Kranjčec, B, D Papeš, and S Altarac. "D-mannose powder for prophylaxis of recurrent urinary tract infections in women: a randomized clinical trial". *World J Urol.* 2014 Feb;32(1):79-84.

26. Jorde, R, ST Sollid, J Svarberq, RM Joakimsen, G Grimnes, MY Hutchinson. "Prevention of urinary tract infections with vitamin D supplementation 20,000 IU per week for five years. Results from an RCT including 511 subjects". *Infect Dis (Lond).* 2016 Jun 30:1-6.

27. Stevens, DL, AL Bisno, HF Chambers, et al. "Practice guidelines for the diagnosis and management of skin and soft tissue infections: 2014 update by the Infectious Diseases Society of America". *Clin Infect Dis.* 2014 Jul 15;59(2):147.

28. Jemec, GB. "Clinical practice. Hidradenitis suppurativa". *N Engl J Med.* 2012;366:158.

29. Aksoy, B, A Altaykan-Hapa, D Egemen, F Karagöz, N Atakan. "The impact of rosacea on quality of life: effects of

demographic and clinical characteristics and various treatment modalities". *Br J Dermatol.* 2010 Oct;163(4):719-725.

30. Liu, C, A Bayer, SE Cosgrove, et al. "Clinical Practice Guidelines by the Infectious Diseases Society of America for the Treatment of methicillin-resistant Staphylococcus aureus infections in adults and children". *Clin Infect Dis.* 2011 Feb 1;52(3):318-355.

Chapter 5

1. Diemert, David J. "Prevention and Self-Treatment of Traveler's Diarrhea". *Clin Microbiol Rev.* July 2006;19(3):583–594.

2. Neal, Keith R, Helen M Scott, Richard S B Slack, Richard F A Logan. "Omeprazole as a risk factor for campylobacter gastroenteritis: case-control study". *BMJ.* 1996;312:414-415.

3. Biswal, S. "Proton pump inhibitors and risk for Clostridium difficile associated diarrhea". *Biomed J.* 2014 Jul-Aug;37(4):178-183.

Chapter 6

1. Katayama, Y, T Inaba, C Nito, and M Ueda. "Neuroprotective effects of erythromycin on ischemic injury following permanent focal cerebral ischemia in rats". *Neurol Res.* 2016 Mar;38(3)275-284. Epub 2016 Mar 16.

2. Zabad, RK, LM Metz, TR Todoruk, Y Zhang, et al. "The clinical response to minocycline in multiple sclerosis is accompanied by beneficial immune changes: a pilot study". *Mult Scler.* 2007 May;13(4):517-526.

3. Bonelli, RM, AK Hödl, P Hofmann, and HP Kapfhammer. "Neuroprotection in Huntington's disease: a 2-year study on minocycline". *Int Clin Psychopharmacol.* 2004 Nov;19(6):337-342.

4. Metchnikoff, Elie, *The Nature of Man, Studies in Optimistic Philosophy*. The Knickerbocker Press, Oct 1903. Reprinted by Forgotten Books (2012).

5. Wirtz, HS, DS Buist, JR Gralow, WE Barlow, et al. "Frequent antibiotic use and second breast cancer events". *Cancer Epidemiol Biomarkers Prev.* 2013 Sep;22(9):1588-1599.

6. Tamim, HM, JA Hanley, AH Hajeer, JF Boivin, JP Collet. "Risk of breast cancer in relation to antibiotic use". *Pharmacoepidemiol Drug Saf.* 2008 Feb;17(2):144-150.

7. Velicer PhD, Christine M, Susan R Heckbert MD, PhD, Johanna W Lampe PhD, RD, John D Potter MD, PhD, Carol A Robertson RPh, Stephen H Taplin MD, MPH. "Antibiotic Use in Relation to the Risk of Breast Cancer". *JAMA.* 2004 Feb 18;291(7):827-835.

8. Lamb, Rebecca, Bela Ozsvari, Camilla L Lisanti, Herbert B Tanowitz, et al. "Antibiotics that target mitochondria effectively eradicate cancer stem cells, across multiple tumor types: Treating cancer like an infectious disease". *Oncotarget.* Jan 2015;6(7):4569-4584.

9. Mellon, Margaret, Karen Lutz Benbrook, and Charles Benbrook. *Hogging It: Estimates of Antimicrobial Abuse in Livestock.* Cambridge, MA: Union of Concerned Scientists. January 2001.

10. Tian, Baoyu, Nibal H Fadhil, J Elijah Powell, Waldan K Kwong, Nancy A Moran. "Long-Term Exposure to Antibiotics Has Caused Accumulation of Resistance Determinants in the Gut Microbiota of Honeybees". *mBio* 30 October 2012;3(6):e00377-12.

11. Peterson, SM, Graeme E Batley, and MS Scammell. "Tetracycline in Antifouling Paints". *Marine Pollution Bulletin.* Feb 1993;26(2):96-100.

12. Garcia, Ahiza. "Sherwin-Williams says new paint will kill bacteria". *CNN Money*. October 31, 2015.

13. Luther PhD, Marla. "Report of FY 2010 Nationwide Survey of Distillers Products for Antibiotic Residues". *Center for Veterinary Medicine, FDA* http://www.fda.gov/ AnimalVeterinary/Products/AnimalFoodFeeds/Contaminants/ ucm300126.htm.

14. Meek, Richard William, Hrushi Vyas, and Laura Jane Violet Piddock. "Nonmedical Uses of Antibiotics: Time to Restrict Their Use?" *PLoS Biol*. October 7, 2015;13(10):e1002266.

Chapter 7

1. Lewis, Kim. "Platforms for antibiotic discovery". *Nature Reviews Drug Discovery*. 2013;12, 371–387.

2. Penicillin VK prescribing information. Sandoz, 2007.

3. Pelton, Ross, J LaValle, EB Hawkins, et al. *Drug Induced Nutrient Depletion Handbook*. Hudson, OH: LexiComp, Inc. 2001:374-385.

4. Augmentin prescribing information. GlaxoSmithKline, 2011.

5. Unasyn prescribing information. Pfizer, 2012.

6. Zosyn prescribing information. Pfizer, 2012.

Chapter 8

1. Campagna, JD, MC Bond, E Schabelman, and BD Hayes. "The use of cephalosporins in penicillin-allergic patients: a literature review". *J Emerg Med*. 2012 May;42(5):612-620.

2. Porter, Robert S. *The Merck Manual* 19th Edition. Merck, 2011.

3. Business Insights. "The Antibacterials Market Outlook to 2016: Competitive landscape, pipeline analysis, and growth opportunities". *Business Insights LTD*. May 2011.

4. Duricef prescribing information. Warner Chilcott Inc, last revised 3 May 2007.

5. Cefazolin prescribing information. West-Ward Pharmaceutical Corp, last revised 8 October 2014.

6. Khawcharoenporn, T and A Tice. "Empiric outpatient therapy with trimethoprim-sulfamethoxazole, cephalexin, or clindamycin for cellulitis". *Am J Med*. 2010 Oct;123(10):942-950.

7. Rajendran, PM, D Young, T Maurer, H Chambers, F Perdreau-Remington, P Ro, H Harris. "Randomized, double-blind, placebo-controlled trial of cephalexin for treatment of uncomplicated skin abscesses in a population at risk for community-acquired methicillin-resistant Staphylococcus aureus infection". *Antimicrob Agents Chemother*. 2007 Nov;51(11):4044-4048.

8. Curtin, CD, JR Casey, PC Murray, CT Cleary, et al. "Efficacy of cephalexin two vs. three times daily vs. cefadroxil once daily for streptococcal tonsillopharyngitis". *Clin Pediatr (Phila)*. 2003 Jul-Aug;42(6):519-526.

9. Cefuroxime package insert. Apotex Corp, last revised 20 July 2015.

10. Cefaclor package insert. Pack Pharmaceuticals, updated Oct 2012.

11. Odio, Carla M, Helen Kusmiesz, Sharon Shelton, John D Nelson. "Comparative treatment trial of augmentin versus cefaclor for acute otitis media with effusion". *Pediatrics*. May 1, 1985;75(5):819-826.

12. Aggarwal, M, R Sinha, MV Murali, P Trihan, PK Singhal.

"Comparative efficacy and safety evaluation of cefaclor vs amoxycillin + clavulanate in children with Acute Otitis Media (AOM)". *Indian J Pediatr*. 2005 Mar;72(3):233-238.

13. Petitpretz, P, C Choné, F Trémolières, and Investigator Study Group. "Levofloxacin 500 mg once daily versus cefuroxime 250 mg twice daily in patients with acute exacerbations of chronic obstructive bronchitis: clinical efficacy and exacerbation-free interval". *Int J Antimicrob Agents*. 2007 Jul;30(1):52-59.

14. Zilinskas, Raymond A. *Biological Warfare: Modern Offense and Defense*. Lynne Rienner Publishers, 2000.

15. Suprax prescribing information. Lupin Pharmaceuticals, revised Oct 2008.

16. Allen, Vanessa G, et al. "Neisseria gonorrhoeae treatment failure and susceptibility to cefixime in Toronto, Canada". *JAMA*. 2013 Jan 9;309(2):163-170.

17. Cefdinir prescribing information. Lupin Pharmaceuticals, revised Dec 2009.

18. Pelton, Ross, J LaValle, EB Hawkins, et al. *Drug Induced Nutrient Depletion Handbook*. Hudson, OH: LexiComp, Inc. 2001:374-385.

Chapter 9

1. Nelson, Mark L, Andrew Dinardo, Jeffrey Hochberg, and George J Armelagos. "Brief communication: Mass spectroscopic characterization of tetracycline in the skeletal remains of an ancient population from Sudanese Nubia 350–550 CE". *American Journal of Physical Anthropology*. September 2010;143(1):151–154.

2. Nagarakanti, Sandhya, Eliahu Bishburg. "Is Minocycline an Anti-Viral Agent? A Review of Current literature". *Basic Clin Pharmacol Toxicol*. Jan 2016;118(1):4-8.

3. Weinberg, JM. "The anti-inflammatory effects of tetracyclines". *Cutis*. 2005 Apr;75(4 Suppl):6-11.

4. Loeb, MB, et al. "A randomized, controlled trial of doxycycline and rifampin for patients with Alzheimer's disease". *J Am Geriatr Soc*. 2004 Mar;52(3):381-387.

5. Seidlitz MSc, Eric, Zeina Saikali PhD, and Gurmit Singh PhD. "Use of Tetracyclines for Bone Metastases" chapter 17 in *Cancer Drug Discovery and Development* (pp 293-303). Springer Link publishers, 2005.

6. Pelton, Ross, J LaValle, EB Hawkins, et al. *Drug Induced Nutrient Depletion Handbook*. Hudson, OH: LexiComp, Inc. 2001:374-385.

7. Doxycycline label. Hikma pharmaceuticals, 2009.

8. Wardyn, SE, et al. "Swine Farming Is a Risk Factor for Infection With and High Prevalence of Carriage of Multidrug-Resistant Staphylococcus aureus". *Clin Infect Dis*. 2015 Jul 1;61(1):59-66.

Chapter 10

1. Hibionada, Florence F. "Remembering the battle of Dr. Abelardo Aguilar: Cure for millions, deprived of millions". The News Today (Accessed on Aug 1, 2015). http://www.thenewstoday.info/2005/05/03/iloilonews3.htm.

2. Xu, Ze-Qi, Michael T Flavin, and David A Eiznhamer. "Chapter 6: Macrolides and Ketolides" in *Antibiotic Discovery and Development: Vol. 1* (pp 181-228). Springer Science & Business Media, 2012.

3. Amsden. GW. "Anti-inflammatory effects of macrolides—an underappreciated benefit in the treatment of community-acquired respiratory tract infections and chronic inflammatory

pulmonary conditions?". *J of Antimicrob Chemother*. (2005) Jan;55(1):10-21.

4. Zithromax data sheet. Pfizer, updated May 2015

5. Biaxin package insert. Abbot Labs, revised July 2012

6. ERYC package insert. Pfizer, 2014

7. Ross MD, PhD, David B. "The FDA and the Case of Ketek". *N Engl J Med*. 2007;356:1601-1604.

8. Ketek prescribing information. Sanofi-Aventis, 2010

9. Williamson, IG, K Rumsby, S Benge, M Moore, PW Smith, M Cross, P Little. "Antibiotics and topical nasal steroid for treatment of acute maxillary sinusitis: a randomized controlled trial". *JAMA*. 2007 Dec 5;298(21):2487-2496.

10. Watkins, RR and TL Lemonovich. "Diagnosis and Management of Community-Acquired Pneumonia in Adults." *Am Fam Physician*. 2011 Jun 1;83(11):1299-1306.

Chapter 11

1. Mingeot-Leclercq, MP, Y Glupczynski, and P Tulkns. "Aminoglycosides: activity and resistance". *Antimicrob Agents Chemother*. 1999 Apr;43(4):727–737

2. Pringle, Peter. *Experiment Eleven: Dark Secrets Behind the Discovery of a Wonder Drug*. Bloomsbury, 2013.

3. Wallgren, A. "Award Presentation Speech". *Nobel Lectures, Physiology or Medicine 1942-1962*. Elsevier, 1964.

4. Waksman, Selman A. "Streptomycin: Background, Isolation, Properties, and Utilization". *Nobel Lectures, Physiology or Medicine 1942-1962*. Elsevier, 1964.

5. Gentamcin product monograph. Baxter, revised 2012.

6. Tobramycin package insert. Pfizer, 2011.

7. Pelton, Ross, J LaValle, EB Hawkins, et al. *Drug Induced Nutrient Depletion Handbook*. Hudson, OH: LexiComp, Inc. 2001:374-385.

8. TOBI inhaler product information. Novartis, March 2015.

9. Tobrex ophlamological ointment package insert. Bausch & Lomb, revised August 2007.

10. Wilschanski MD, Michael, et al. "Gentamicin-Induced Correction of CFTR Function in Patients with Cystic Fibrosis and *CFTR* Stop Mutations". *N Engl J Med*. 2003;349:1433–1441.

Chapter 12

1. "Gerhard Domagk Biography". *Nobel Lectures, Physiology or Medicine 1922-1941*. Elsevier Publishing,1965.

2. Borkin, Joseph. *The Crime and Punishment of I.G. Farben*. Free Press, 1978.

3. Bactrim prescribing information. Roche, revised March 2015.

4. Septra drug label. Monarch Pharmaceuticals, September 2006.

5. Pelton, Ross, J LaValle, EB Hawkins, et al. *Drug Induced Nutrient Depletion Handbook*. Hudson, OH: LexiComp, Inc. 2001:374-385.

6. Ballentine, C. "Taste of Raspberries, Taste of Death: The 1937 Elixir Sulfanilamide Incident". *FDA Consumer magazine*. June 1981 Issue.

7. Harris, R. "China's Unwatched Drug Makers". *NY Times*. October 31, 2007. http://www.nytimes.com/video/world/1194817122573/china-s-unwatched-drug-makers.html

Chapter 13

1. Andriole, Vincent T. "The quinolones: past, present, and future". *Clin Infect Dis.* 2005 Jul 15;41 Suppl 2: S113-S119. (Nalidixic acid was not much used in the 1960s because there was not yet a widespread problem with bacterial resistance to other, less toxic drugs.)

2. "OEHHA Prop 65 List" – California Office of Environmental Health Hazard Assessment List as required by The California Safe Drinking Water and Toxic Enforcement Act of 1986.

3. Xia, Y, ZY Yang, SL Morris-Natschke, and KH Lee. "Recent advances in the discovery and development of quinolones and analogs as antitumor agents". *Curr Med Chem.* 1999 Mar;6(3):179-194.

4. Mandell, Lewis, and Glenn S Tillotson. "Safety of Fluoroquinolones: An Update". *The Canadian Journal of Infectious Diseases.* Feb 2002;13(1):54–61.

5. Nelson, Jennifer M, Tom M Chiller, John H Powers, and Frederick J Angulo. "Fluoroquinolone-resistant Campylobacter species and the withdrawal of fluoroquinolones from use in poultry: a public health success story". *Clin Infect Dis.* 2007 Apr 1;44(7):977-980.

6. Fried, Stephen. *Bitter Pills: Inside the Hazardous World of Legal Drugs.* Bantam 2011.

7. Cipro package insert. Bayer (manufacturer) and Schering Plough (distributor), 2015.

8. Levaquin package insert. Patriot Pharmaceuticals, 2013.

9. Pelton, Ross, J LaValle, EB Hawkins, et al. *Drug Induced Nutrient Depletion Handbook.* Hudson, OH: LexiComp, Inc. 2001:374-385.

Chapter 14

1. Flagyl package insert. Pfizer, 2016.

2. Bahmani, M, K Saki, M Rafieian-Kopaei, SA Karamati, Z Eftekhari, M Jelodari. "The most common herbal medicines affecting Sarcomastigophora branches: a review study". *Asian Pac J Trop Med.* 2014 Sep;7S1:S14-21.

3. Ware, Elinor. "The Chemistry of the Hydantoins". *Chem Rev.* June 1950;46(3):403-470.

4. United States. Congress. "Office of Technology Assessment: *Drugs in livestock feed (1979)* Volume 1: Technical Report". DIANE Publishing, 1979.

5. Phongvivat, Sujittra. "Nitrofurans Case Study: Thailand's experience." Joint FAO/WHO Technical Workshop on Working Paper: Residues of Substances without ADI/MRL in Food. Bangkok, 24. – 26.8. 2004.

6. US FDA Import Alert 16-129: "Detention Without Physical Examination of Seafood Products Due to Nitrofurans". *US FDA.* 11/20/2015.

7. Macrodantin package insert. Procter & Gamble Pharmaceuticals, 2009.

8. Xifaxan package insert. Salix Inc, 2015.

9. Vancomycin package insert. Sandoz, 2015.

10. Zyvox package insert. Pfizer, 2015.

11. Department of Justice, Office of Public Affairs Press Release: "Justice Department Announces Largest Health Care Fraud Settlement in Its History: Pfizer to Pay $2.3 Billion for Fraudulent Marketing". September 2, 2009. http://www.justice.gov/opa/pr/justice-department-announces-largest-health-care-fraud-settlement-its-history.

12. Neu, HC, A Prince, CO Neu, and GJ Garvey. "Incidence of diarrhea and colitis associated with clindamycin therapy". *J Infect Dis*. 1977 Mar;135 Suppl:S120-125.

13. Cleocin package insert. Pfizer, October 2013.

14. Global Tuberculosis Control 2012, WHO, Geneva, 2012.

15. Paser package insert. Jacobus Pharmaceutical Company Inc, 2010.

16. Wang, Feng, Robert Langley, Gulcin Gulten, Lynn G Dover, et al. "Mechanism of thioamide drug action against tuberculosis and leprosy". *J Exper Med*. Jan 2007;204(1):73-78.

17. Cycloserine drug label. Purdue, 2011.

18. Karlock DPM, Lawrence. "What You Should Know About Using Silver Products in Wound Care". *Podiatry Today*. Nov 2004;17(11).

19. Carter, DA, SE Blair, NN Cokcetin, D Bouzo, P Brooks, R Schothauer, EJ Harry. "Therapeutic Manuka Honey: No Longer So Alternative". *Front Microbiol*. 2016 Apr 20;7:569.

20. Reuter, J, I Merfort, CM Schempp. "Botanicals in dermatology: an evidence-based review". *Am J Clin Dermatol*. 2010;11(4):247-267.

Chapter 15

1. Ruiz, Rebecca. "Ten Misleading Drug Ads". Posted 2/02/2010 on Forbes.com. http://www.forbes.com/2010/02/02/drug-advertising-lipitor-lifestyle-health-pharmaceuticals-safety.html.

2. Smith, Richard. "Medical Journals Are an Extension of the Marketing Arm of Pharmaceutical Companies". *PLoS Med*. May 2005;2(5):e138.

DRUG INDEX

Achromycin (see Tetracyclines)

Acuatim (see Quinolones – The "Floxin" Drugs)

Amikacin (see Aminoglycosides)

Amikin (see Aminoglycosides)

Aminoglycosides

Amoxicillin (see Penicillins)

Amoxil (see Penicillins)

Ampicillin (see Penicillins)

Ancef (see Cephalosporins)

Avelox (see Quinolones – The "Floxin" Drugs)

Avycaz (see Cephalosporins and Penicillins)

Azelaic acid (see Miscellaneous Antibiotics)

Azithromycin (see Macrolides (Erythromycin and Related Drugs))

Bacampicillin (see Penicillins)

Baciguent (see Miscellaneous Antibiotics)

Bacitracin (see Miscellaneous Antibiotics)

Bactocill (see Penicillins)

Bactrim (see Sulfa Drugs)

Bactrim DS (see Sulfa Drugs)

Balofloxacin (see Quinolones – The "Floxin" Drugs)

Baloxin (see Quinolones – The "Floxin" Drugs)

Beepen-VK (see Penicillins)

Besifloxacin (see Quinolones – The "Floxin" Drugs)

Besivance (see Quinolones – The "Floxin" Drugs)

Betapen-VK (see Penicillins)

Biaxin (see Macrolides (Erythromycin and Related Drugs))

Bicillin L-A (see Penicillins)

carbapenems. (see Penicillins)

Carbenicillin (see Penicillins)

Ceclor (see Cephalosporins)

Ceclor CD (see Cephalosporins)

Cedax (see Cephalosporins)

Cefacetrile (see Cephalosporins)

Cefaclomezine (see Cephalosporins)

Cefaclor (see Cephalosporins)

Cefadroxil (see Cephalosporins)

Cefadroxyl (see Cephalosporins)

Cefadyl (see Cephalosporins)

Cefalexin (see Cephalosporins)

Cefaloglycin (see Cephalosporins)

Cefalonium (see Cephalosporins)

Cefaloram (see Cephalosporins)

Cefaloridine (see Cephalosporins)

Cefalotin (see Cephalosporins)

Cefamandol (see Cephalosporins)

Cefaparole (see Cephalosporins)

Cefapirin (see Cephalosporins)

Cefatrizine (see Cephalosporins)

Cefazaflur (see Cephalosporins)

Cefazedone (see Cephalosporins)

Cefazolin (see Cephalosporins)

Cefcanel (see Cephalosporins)

Cefcapene (see Cephalosporins)

Cefclidine (see Cephalosporins)

Cefdaloxime (see Cephalosporins)

Cefdiel (see Cephalosporins)

Cefdinir (see Cephalosporins)

Cefditoren (see Cephalosporins)

Cefedrolor (see Cephalosporins)

Cefempidone (see Cephalosporins)

Cefepime (see Cephalosporins)

Cefetamet (see Cephalosporins)

Cefetrizole (see Cephalosporins)

Cefivitril (see Cephalosporins)

Cefixime (see Cephalosporins)

Cefizox (see Cephalosporins)

Cefluprenam (see Cephalosporins)

Cefmatilen (see Cephalosporins)

Cefmax (see Cephalosporins)

Cefmenoxime (see Cephalosporins)

Cefmepidium (see Cephalosporins)

Cefmetazole (see Cephalosporins)

Cefobid (see Cephalosporins)

Cefodizime (see Cephalosporins)

Cefonicid (see Cephalosporins)

Cefoperazone (see Cephalosporins)

Cefoselis (see Cephalosporins)

Cefotan (see Cephalosporins)

Cefotaxime (see Cephalosporins)

Cefotetan (see Cephalosporins)

Cefovecin (see Cephalosporins)

Cefoxazole (see Cephalosporins)

Cefoxitin (see Cephalosporins)

Cefozopran (see Cephalosporins)

Cefpimizole (see Cephalosporins)

Cefpirome (see Cephalosporins)

Cefpodoxime (see Cephalosporins)

cefproxil (see Cephalosporins)

Cefprozil (see Cephalosporins)

Cefquinome (see Cephalosporins)

Cefradine (see Cephalosporins)

Cefrom (see Cephalosporins)

Cefrotil (see Cephalosporins)

Cefroxadine (see Cephalosporins)

Cefsumide (see Cephalosporins)

Ceftaroline (see Cephalosporins)

Ceftazidime (see Cephalosporins)

Ceftazidime/Avibactam (see Cephalosporins and Penicillins)

Cefteram (see Cephalosporins)

Ceftezole (see Cephalosporins)

Ceftibuten (see Cephalosporins)

Ceftin (see Cephalosporins)

Ceftiofur (see Cephalosporins)

Ceftiolene (see Cephalosporins)

Ceftioxide (see Cephalosporins)

Ceftizoxime (see Cephalosporins)

Ceftobiprole (see Cephalosporins)

Ceftriaxone (see Cephalosporins)

Cefuracetime (see Cephalosporins)

Cefuroxime (see Cephalosporins)

Cefuzonam (see Cephalosporins)

Cefzil (see Cephalosporins)

Celospor (see Cephalosporins)

Celtol (see Cephalosporins)

Cephacetrile (see Cephalosporins)

cephalexin (see Cephalosporins)

cephaloglycin (see Cephalosporins)

cephalonium) (see Cephalosporins)

cephaloradine (see Cephalosporins)

Cephalosporins

cephalothin (see Cephalosporins)

cephapirin (see Cephalosporins)

cephazolin (see Cephalosporins)

cephradine (see Cephalosporins)

Ceptaz (see Cephalosporins)

Chloramphenicol (see Traveler's Diarrhea)

Cipro (see Quinolones – The "Floxin" Drugs)

Cipro XR (see Quinolones – The "Floxin" Drugs)

Ciprobay (see Quinolones – The "Floxin" Drugs)

Ciprofloxacin (see Quinolones – The "Floxin" Drugs)

Ciproxin (see Quinolones – The "Floxin" Drugs)

Claforan (see Cephalosporins)

Clarithromycin (see Macrolides (Erythromycin and Related Drugs))

Cleocin (see Lincosamides)

Clinafloxacin (see Quinolones – The "Floxin" Drugs)

Clindamycin (see Lincosamides)

Cloxacillin (see Penicillins)

Cloxapen (see Penicillins)

Cotrim (see Sulfa Drugs)

Cotrim DS (see Sulfa Drugs)

Cravit (see Quinolones – The "Floxin" Drugs)

Cristacef (see Cephalosporins)

Crysticillin 300 A.S. (see Penicillins)

Cubicin (see Daptomycin)

Cycloserine (see Miscellaneous Antibiotics)

Daptomycin

Declomycin (see Tetracyclines)

Demeclocycline (see Tetracyclines)

Dicloxacillin (see Penicillins)

Dirithromycin (see Macrolides (Erythromycin and Related Drugs))

Distaclor (see Cephalosporins)

Dolcol (see Quinolones – The "Floxin" Drugs)

Doryx (see Tetracyclines)

Doxycycline (see Tetracyclines)

Duricef (see Cephalosporins)

Dycill (see Penicillins)

Dynabac (see Macrolides (Erythromycin and Related Drugs))

Dynacin (see Tetracyclines)

Dynapen (see Penicillins)

Enoxacin (see Quinolones – The "Floxin" Drugs)

Enroxil (see Quinolones – The "Floxin" Drugs)

Eradacil (see Quinolones – The "Floxin" Drugs)

Erythromycin (see Macrolides (Erythromycin and Related Drugs))

Ethambutol (see Miscellaneous Antibiotics)

Ethionamide (see Miscellaneous Antibiotics)

Excede (see Cephalosporins)

Factive (see Quinolones – The "Floxin" Drugs)

Factive (see Quinolones – The "Floxin" Drugs)

Flagyl (see Miscellaneous Antibiotics)

Flopen (see Penicillins)

Flopen (see Penicillins)

Flopen (see Penicillins)

Floxapen (see Penicillins)

Floxin (see Quinolones – The "Floxin" Drugs)

Flubactin (see Quinolones – The "Floxin" Drugs)

Flucloxacillin (see Penicillins)

Flumequine (see Quinolones – The "Floxin" Drugs)

Fluoroquinolones

Fortaz (see Cephalosporins)

Fortum (see Cephalosporins)

Furadantin (see Miscellaneous Antibiotics)

G-Mycin (see Aminoglycosides)

Gantanol (see Sulfa Drugs)

Gantrisin (see Sulfa Drugs)

Garamycin (see Aminoglycosides)

Gatifloxacin (see Quinolones – The "Floxin" Drugs)

Gemifloxacin (see Quinolones – The "Floxin" Drugs)

Gemifloxacin (see Quinolones – The "Floxin" Drugs)

Gentamicin (see Aminoglycosides)

Geocillin (see Penicillins)

Geopen (see Penicillins)

Glycylcyclines (see Tetracyclines)

Gracevit (see Quinolones – The "Floxin" Drugs)

Grepafloxacin (see Quinolones – The "Floxin" Drugs)

INH (see Miscellaneous Antibiotics)

Isoniazid (see Miscellaneous Antibiotics)

Ivermectin topical (see Miscellaneous Antibiotics)

Janacin (see Quinolones – The "Floxin" Drugs)

Jenamicin (see Aminoglycosides)

Kanamycin (see Aminoglycosides)

Kantrex (see Aminoglycosides)

Kefglycin (see Cephalosporins)

Keflex (see Cephalosporins)

Keflin (see Cephalosporins)

Keflor (see Cephalosporins)

Keftab (see Cephalosporins)

Kefurox (see Cephalosporins)

Kefzol (see Cephalosporins)

Ketek (see Macrolides (Erythromycin and Related Drugs))

Ketolides (see Macrolides (Erythromycin and Related Drugs))

Ledercillin VK (see Penicillins)

Levaquin (see Quinolones – The "Floxin" Drugs)

Levofloxacin (see Quinolones – The "Floxin" Drugs)

Lexinor (see Quinolones – The "Floxin" Drugs)

Lincocin (see Lincosamides)

Lincomycin (see Lincosamides)

Lincosamides

Lipopeptides (see Daptomycin)

Lomefloxacin (see Quinolones – The "Floxin" Drugs)

Macrobid (see Miscellaneous Antibiotics)

Macrodantin (see Miscellaneous Antibiotics)

Macrolides (Erythromycin and Related Drugs)

Mandol (see Cephalosporins)

Maxaquin (see Quinolones – The "Floxin" Drugs)

Maxipime (see Cephalosporins)

Mefoxin (see Cephalosporins)

Metronidazole (see Miscellaneous Antibiotics)

Mezlin (see Penicillins)

Mezlocillin (see Penicillins)

Minocin (see Tetracyclines)

Minocycline (see Tetracyclines)

Monobactams (see Penicillins)

Monocid (see Cephalosporins)

Monodox (see Tetracyclines)

Moxifloxacin (see Quinolones – The "Floxin" Drugs)

Mycifradin (see Aminoglycosides)

Myciguent (see Aminoglycosides)

Nadifloxacin (see Quinolones – The "Floxin" Drugs)

Nadixa (see Quinolones – The "Floxin" Drugs)

Nadoxin (see Quinolones – The "Floxin" Drugs)

Nafcil (see Penicillins)

Nafcillin (see Penicillins)

Nalidixic acid (see Quinolones – The "Floxin" Drugs)

Nallpen (see Penicillins)

Nebcin (see Aminoglycosides)

NegGam (see Quinolones – The "Floxin" Drugs)

Neomycin (see Aminoglycosides)

Neosprin (see Miscellaneous Antibiotics)

Netilmicin (see Aminoglycosides)

Netromycin (see Aminoglycosides)

Nitrofurantoin (see Miscellaneous Antibiotics)

Norfloxacin (see Quinolones – The "Floxin" Drugs)

Noroxin (see Quinolones – The "Floxin" Drugs)

Ofloxacin (see Quinolones – The "Floxin" Drugs)

Omnicef (see Cephalosporins)

Omniflox (see Quinolones – The "Floxin" Drugs)

Omnipen (see Penicillins)

Oxacillin (see Penicillins)

Oxaldin (see Quinolones – The "Floxin" Drugs)

Oxolinic acid (see Quinolones – The "Floxin" Drugs)

Oxytetracycline (see Tetracyclines)

Ozex (see Quinolones – The "Floxin" Drugs)

Panacid (see Quinolones – The "Floxin" Drugs)

Para-aminosalicylic acid (see Miscellaneous Antibiotics)

Paromomycin (see Aminoglycosides)

PASER (see Miscellaneous Antibiotics)

Pasil (see Quinolones – The "Floxin" Drugs)

Pathocil (see Penicillins)

Pazucross (see Quinolones – The "Floxin" Drugs)

Pazufloxacin (see Quinolones – The "Floxin" Drugs)

Peflacine (see Quinolones – The "Floxin" Drugs)

Pefloxacin (see Quinolones – The "Floxin" Drugs)

Penetrex (see Quinolones – The "Floxin" Drugs)

Penicillins

Penicillin G (see Penicillins)

Penicillin V (see Penicillins)

Pentids (see Penicillins)

Permapen (see Penicillins)

Pfizerpen (see Penicillins)

Pfizerpen-AS (see Penicillins)

Pipemidic acid (see Quinolones – The "Floxin" Drugs)

Piperacillin (see Penicillins)

Pipracil (see Penicillins)

Piromidic acid (see Quinolones – The "Floxin" Drugs)

Pivampicillin (see Penicillins)

Pivmecillinam (see Penicillins)

Polycillin (see Penicillins)

Polycillin-N (see Penicillins)

Polymox (see Penicillins)

Polymyxin B (see Miscellaneous Antibiotics)

Principen (see Penicillins)

Prostaphlin (see Penicillins)

Protionamide (see Miscellaneous Antibiotics)

Prulifloxacin (see Quinolones – The "Floxin" Drugs)

Pyrazinamide (see Miscellaneous Antibiotics)

Quinabic (see Quinolones – The "Floxin" Drugs)

Quinolones – The "Floxin" Drugs

Quisnon (see Quinolones – The "Floxin" Drugs)

Ranicor (see Cephalosporins)

Raxar (see Quinolones – The "Floxin" Drugs)

Rifampicin (see Miscellaneous Antibiotics)

Rifampin (see Miscellaneous Antibiotics)

Rocephin (see Cephalosporins)

Rosoxacin (see Quinolones – The "Floxin" Drugs)

Roxithromycin (see Macrolides (Erythromycin and Related Drugs))

Rufloxacin (see Quinolones – The "Floxin" Drugs)

Rulid (see Macrolides (Erythromycin and Related Drugs))

Septra (see Sulfa Drugs)

Septra DS (see Sulfa Drugs)

Sitafloxacin (see Quinolones – The "Floxin" Drugs)

Sparfloxacin (see Quinolones – The "Floxin" Drugs)

Spectracef (see Cephalosporins)

Spectrobid (see Penicillins)

Staphcillin (see Penicillins)

Streptomycin (see Aminoglycosides)

Sulfacetamide-sulfur (see Miscellaneous Antibiotics)

Sulfamethizole (see Sulfa Drugs)

Sulfamethoxazole (see Sulfa Drugs)

Sulfatrim (see Sulfa Drugs)

Sulfatrim-DS (see Sulfa Drugs)

Sulfisoxazole (see Sulfa Drugs)

Sulfonamides (see Sulfa Drugs)

Suprax (see Cephalosporins)

Surlid (see Macrolides (Erythromycin and Related Drugs))

Tarivid (see Quinolones – The "Floxin" Drugs)

Tazicef (see Cephalosporins)

Tazidime (see Cephalosporins)

Teflaro (see Cephalosporins)

Telithromycin (see Macrolides (Erythromycin and Related Drugs))

Temafloxacin (see Quinolones – The "Floxin" Drugs)

Tequin (see Quinolones – The "Floxin" Drugs)

Terizidone (see Miscellaneous Antibiotics)

Terramycin (see Tetracyclines)

Tetracyclines

Thinamide (see Miscellaneous Antibiotics)

Thiosulfil Forte (see Sulfa Drugs)

Ticar (see Penicillins)

Ticarcillin (see Penicillins)

Tigecycline (see Tetracyclines)

Tobramycin (see Aminoglycosides)

Tosacin (see Quinolones – The "Floxin" Drugs)

Tosufloxacin (see Quinolones – The "Floxin" Drugs)

Totacillin (see Penicillins)

Trimethoprim-Sulfamethoxazole (see Sulfa Drugs)

Trimox (see Penicillins)

Triple Antibiotic Ointment (see Miscellaneous Antibiotics)

Trovafloxacin (see Quinolones – The "Floxin" Drugs)

Trovan (see Quinolones – The "Floxin" Drugs)

Tygacil (see Tetracyclines)

Ultracef (see Cephalosporins)

Unipen (see Penicillins)

Urobak (see Sulfa Drugs)

Uroflox (see Quinolones – The "Floxin" Drugs)

Uroxin (see Quinolones – The "Floxin" Drugs)

V-Cillin K (see Penicillins)

Vancocin (see Miscellaneous Antibiotics)

Vancomycin (see Miscellaneous Antibiotics)

Vantin (see Cephalosporins)

Velosef (see Cephalosporins)

Vibramycin (see Tetracyclines)

Vigamox (see Quinolones – The "Floxin" Drugs)

Wintomylon (see Quinolones – The "Floxin" Drugs)

Wycillin (see Penicillins)

Wymox (see Penicillins)

Zagam (see Quinolones – The "Floxin" Drugs)

Zeftera (see Cephalosporins)

Zinacef (see Cephalosporins)

Zinnat (see Cephalosporins)

Zithromax (see Macrolides (Erythromycin and Related Drugs))

Zymar (see Quinolones – The "Floxin" Drugs)

www.ingramcontent.com/pod-product-compliance
Lightning Source LLC
Chambersburg PA
CBHW050727030426
42336CB00012B/1451